THE LIFE OF BRIAN
CONFESSIONS OF AN OLYMPIC DOCTOR

BRIAN CORRIGAN

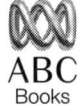
ABC Books

Published by ABC Books for the
AUSTRALIAN BROADCASTING CORPORATION
GPO Box 9994 Sydney NSW 2001

Copyright © Dr Brian Corrigan and Malcolm Andrews 2004

First published August 2004

All rights reserved. No part of this publication may be reproduced, stored in a retrieval system or transmitted in any form or by any means, electronic, mechanical, photocopying, recording or otherwise, without the prior written permission of the Australian Broadcasting Corporation.

National Library of Australia
Cataloguing-in-Publication data:
    Corrigan, Brian, 1915-
    The life of Brian : confessions of an Olympic doctor.

    Includes bibliographical references and index.
    ISBN 0 7333 1443 0.

    1. Corrigan, Brian, 1915-. 2. Sports medicine. 3. Medicine - Specialties and specialists - Australia. 4. Rheumatologists - Australia - Biography. I. Title.

    617.1027

Cover design by Kerry Klinner
Internals set in 11/15pt Palatino Light by Kirby Jones
Colour reproduction by Colorwize Studio, Adelaide
Printed and bound in Australia by Griffin Press, Adelaide

Dedicated to my six muses:
Monica, Sue Ellen, Carolyn, Shayne,
Joanne and Dominic

ACKNOWLEDGEMENTS

There is no way this book could ever have been finished without the valuable help and expertise of my good friend Malcolm Andrews (aka Malcolm X, although I prefer to call him Ace). He also arranged the nine interviews scattered through this book. Malcolm has worked as a journalist both here and overseas, and so has a wide experience in newspapers, radio and television. He is also the author of some twenty-three books, the most recent being the about the life and times of Kostya Tszyu, while his next book is on Australian trivia. He is now a freelance writer and has just moved to Port Macquarie. Thanks so much, mate.

Next in line for thanks would have to be my publisher, Stuart Neal, and editor, Susan Morris-Yates, at ABC Books for taking a chance on me and for the subsequent patient assistance.

Richie Benaud OBE and Johnny Warren MBE, OAM, both exceedingly busy friends, willingly agreed to write forewords. Thank you.

Thanks to those Corrigans — Dominic, Joanne and Christine — who read the text and supplied constructive criticism. And anyone who knows my wife, Monica, would know I could never function without her.

Others I would like to thank include Raelene Boyle, Ron Clarke, Dr Merv Cross, Alan Davidson AM, MBE, Professor Ken Fitch AM, Alan Jones, Neal Marks, Tim Moore, Julius 'Judy' Patching AO, OBE, Rale Rasic OAM, Joan and Les Symons for their clever suggestion, Alan Trengove, James Valentine and Charlie Yankos.

All my registrars, bright young people, taught me far more than I ever taught them, and had to listen to these stories at least three times without ever seeming to mind.

And finally, to my friend, my daughter Sue Ellen. Only two people realise how great her contribution has been.

It would seem inevitable that I have missed someone out, but if so they will understand that old men forget, as Shakespeare says in *Henry V*, and will forgive me for simply falling prey to the ageing process. I apologise in advance…

CONTENTS

Forewords
    Richie Benaud   1
    John Warren   3
Introduction   5

1. The Kid From Glebe   9
2. A Country Practice   15
3. City Limits   21
4. Cotton's Field   30
5. Making a Reputation   36
6. Quietly Flows the Don   44
7. Nugget of Gold   51
8. Not a Case of Luck   57
9. Richie's Last Ball   62
10. Genius or Ratbag?   75
11. Breathless and Bewildered   80
12. A Broken Heart   86
13. A Great Idea   99
14. The Shattered Dream   107
15. Prime Minister Booed   114
16. Russian Roulette   119
17. Highs and Lows   126
18. If He's from Apia, Pick Him   135
19. The KY to Victory   140
20. Jack the Quack   147
21. The Reluctant Hero   153
22. So Near, Yet So Far   156
23. A Tough Road to Germany   160

24.	A Sporting Tragedy	166
25.	In the Major League	171
26.	Massaging the Spirit	181
27.	The Good, the Bad and the Mad	185
28.	My Friend, the Witch Doctor	195
29.	Blood and Guts	200
30.	Pros and Cons	213
31.	Dame Margot and Sir Bobbie	221
32.	A Mad, Mad World	226
33.	The Cruel Sea	239
34.	A Brain Tumour	242
35.	Sex at the Olympics	253
36.	Pandora's Box	263
37.	Catching the Cheats	270
38.	Sydney 2000 Drug Testing	276
39.	Alternative Medicine	281
40.	Sports' Everest	285
41.	Seven Pillars of Improvement	289
42.	The Genie in the Bottle	293
43.	THG — The Last Menace	297

FOREWORD
By Richie Benaud OBE

THERE ARE ALWAYS good reasons for writing a foreword for a book, although I rarely do so. This one is for a special reason and a good friend; the reason being that my cricket career would have finished and the 1961 Ashes would not have been retained by Australia had Brian Corrigan not been on hand in England at the time. In those days there was normal back-up for a team, nothing like the entourage which accompanies the modern-day Australian touring teams, but good nevertheless.

Brian, a young doctor and sports medicine specialist, was in England studying at the time and although he wasn't at Worcester when I injured a shoulder in the opening match of the tour, he was at Edgbaston for the First Test of the series when I broke down again on the final day.

He phoned me the next morning and we had breakfast together, in the course of which he told me he doubted the treatment I was having at the time would do the job. He recommended a new-style treatment which was successful for injuries of this kind and was being pioneered by Dr Alan Bass, who was the club doctor at Arsenal Football Club.

It was hard work but Alan Bass and his revolutionary ideas had me greatly improved for the two matches leading into the Old Trafford Test, and the celebrations on 1 August 1961, at the Midland Hotel, Manchester, and on the subsequent train journey to London, were some of the sweetest I had experienced.

Not long after that, the last time I captained Australia, was at the 'Gabba Test which finished on 11 December 1963. Ten days later Brian was at Mosman Oval when, in a club match, I dropped a catch off Doug Walters and, after he drove me to hospital, the X-rays confirmed a break in three places in my spinning finger. I said to Brian, 'I don't care how you manage it. I know I can't be fit for the Melbourne Test but I must pass a fitness test and play in the Third Test at the Sydney Cricket Ground.'

'In that case,' he said. 'There's no point in putting it in plaster.' He pulled a squash ball out of the glove box of his car and said, 'There you are. Squeeze that a thousand times a day and you'll be OK.' And I was!

When we were trying to find a way for me to move more freely because of back problems, I had a considerable number of scans and X-rays. When he phoned to say to come over to the surgery I was just a mite apprehensive.

The apprehension was dissipated quickly as each of the X-rays was placed on the glass with the white light behind it, accompanied by delighted and approving murmurs from Dr Corrigan. Calm and confident now I ventured, 'Sounds as though everything is great then — the back is in perfect shape?'

'Heavens, no! It's in the worst shape imaginable, but the convention at which I'm speaking on Tuesday will be enthralled to see what can happen to a cricketer who bowls more than 50,000 balls of over-the-wrist spin in 16 years.'

He was never short of a sense of humour and many years ago I was flying to England and tried to obtain a glass of chardonnay once we had taken off. After the tenth time of asking, and being refused the captain of the plane came down and explained that my family doctor had been in contact to say that Mr Benaud shouldn't be given any alcohol as he was on medication.

Great guy Corrigan, splendid doctor, keen lover of all sport and a very good friend of ours for more than 40 years. I hope this book goes as well as his teaching. He thoroughly deserves it.

FOREWORD
By John Warren MBE, OAM

I WAS FIRST introduced to Brian Corrigan, our new team doctor, in 1967 when the Australian soccer team was playing three matches against Scotland and the NSW team was to play Manchester United. Our coach, the much-loved 'Uncle Joe' Vlasits, told the team that Brian was a specialist in the new field of sports medicine, was going to check us for injuries and also organise a series of fitness tests at the University of Sydney. Nobody had ever taken any interest in such matters before, but what we didn't realise was that the tests turned out to be harder than the training we used to do in those days. Everyone found out just how fit (or unfit) he was, and we felt we were part of this new world of sports medicine.

When growing up in Botany, I played a great deal of cricket and soccer, and possibly even loved cricket then more than soccer. Cricket players, especially dashing ones like Richie Benaud, Norm O'Neill and Doug Walters, were my idols. So I found it difficult to realise that here was the doctor who knew them and treated them all, and I felt suitably impressed.

Everyone coming into a closed community, as a soccer team is, is at first treated with a certain degree of suspicion and reserve. They have to earn the trust of the team. But our doctor seemed so friendly and relaxed — 'She'll be right,' he'd say — and, better still, even seemed to know what he was talking about, that he immediately seemed to fit in, becoming one of the boys and an important part of our team structure. From then on, he was never known by any other name than the Doc. He was to become a legend.

We have remained the best of friends ever since, and he has two characteristics I especially admired. He would always stand up for the player, even though that sometimes would bring him into conflict with the soccer establishment. But he would stick to his guns.

The other was he was such a good tourist. Whenever the going was tough, as it was in Saigon later that year, he was always cheerful, taking the smooth with the rough.

Subsequently, the two of us often toured together with the Australian team, and since we were both interested in the people of the nation we were visiting, whenever there was a rare opportunity to get a day off, we would explore the country together. The one time I particularly treasure was in Israel when we climbed Masada — this mountain is the site of the last Jewish resistance against the Romans, and all who remained committed suicide rather than surrender — and went for a swim in the Dead Sea, where the high salt content allows you to float on the surface.

I would like to add a personal note. Throughout my career, I have had some major injuries, none greater than the ruptured cruciate ligament that threatened my career. In those days, precious little was known about such injuries or their treatment, and I became the first in Australia to have the newly prescribed operation, a knee reconstruction. Rehabilitation was prolonged and intensive, but we were determined to get back on the field. Thankfully, I was able to make it to play in the World Cup in West Germany.

Another time, I had blood poisoning due to an infected knee. Doc had me in hospital and on treatment before I even realised what was going on. One of the doctors at the hospital told me later that that action probably saved my leg and my life.

The story in this book about Brian's recovery from a brain tumour has been a great help to me now I have a problem of my own. Finally, he has also been a great friend of, and doctor to, many members of my family.

The book contains many interesting and amusing anecdotes about some of the amazing characters he has met since those first days, not only from the world of soccer, but also from cricket, the Olympics, and his own medical practice.

It has truly been a great honour to be asked to write a foreword for my very good friend. I wish him and his book every success.

INTRODUCTION

THE HISTORY OF the modern Olympics has been peppered by mistakes by the apparently well-meaning but naive (and often chauvinist) old men of the self-elected International Olympic Committee.

For a start, women weren't allowed to compete in swimming events until 1912, when Australia's Fanny Durack and Mina Wylie finished one–two in the 100-metre freestyle. They weren't allowed on the athletics track until 1928 when they were permitted to compete in the 100-metre sprint and the 800-metre so-called 'endurance event'. When several collapsed after the latter race, the Olympic chiefs in collaboration with the international athletics authorities decided that in future they would be banned from races over distances longer than 200 metre. And so it was for the next 32 years.

They also robbed that wonderful Dutch athlete Fanny Blankers-Koen of a couple of gold medals at the 1948 Olympics by decreeing that no one could compete in more than four events. She won the 100-metre, 200-metre, 80-metre hurdles and was part of the winning 4 x 100-metre relay (in which the Dutch beat the Australians into second place). But Fanny was banned by the IOC from also competing in the high jump and long jump even though she held the world record in both these events.

There was many an occasion that the IOC turned a blind eye to 'shamateurism', the under-the-table payments to allegedly amateur sportsmen and women. Yet their draconian powers meant that Australian diver Dick Eve, a gold medal winner at the 1924 Paris Olympics, was declared to be professional a year later and could not compete in the Olympics again. His only crime was to succeed his father as manager of the Manly Swimming Baths.

What about the IOC's inability to halt the drug-taking of the sportsmen and women from behind the Iron Curtain in the 1970s and beyond? And their failure to rein in the drug cheats of America in recent years?

One of the major regular stuff-ups has been the research — or lack of it — leading to the selection of cities to host the world's ultimate sporting tournament.

There was the choice of Atlanta for the 1996 Games to appease Coca-Cola, one of the Olympics major sponsors, whose world headquarters just happened to be in that city. Montreal was given the Olympics in 1976 even though the figures showed they would be a financial disaster. The unfortunate people of Quebec were still paying off the debt decades later.

But the blunder to trump all blunders was the IOC's decision to hold the 1968 Olympics in Mexico City. There was, of course, the threat of civil unrest, which should have set the alarm bells ringing. But it was the Olympic bosses' decision to ignore the medical warnings of the dire consequences of holding the Games at the high altitude of Mexico City — 2240 metres above sea level — that will remain forever a blight on the record of the old buffers in the IOC.

The warnings were ignored for purely political reasons. The IOC wanted Latin America to host an Olympics come what may. The bungle was exacerbated by the autocratic Olympic chief Avery Brundage who agreed that athletes should be allowed to train at high altitude — but to preserve their amateur status that training was to be restricted to just four weeks in the year preceding the Mexico City Olympics. How blind could one be!

No one died during competition in Mexico City, as one Swedish professor had predicted. But it was more through good luck than planning. In one single day of the Games no less than 18 rowers collapsed. On another, half the competitors in the modern pentathlon suffered a similar fate.

The most dramatic example of the stupidity of the IOC in ignoring the best medical advice in the world was what happened to Australia's champion long distance runner, Ron Clarke. The man who held every world record from 2000 metres to 10,000 metres was reduced to a mere mortal by the high altitude, collapsing in a heap at the end of the 10,000 metres, the first track and field event decided in Mexico City.

There are but a few flickering moments of television coverage and some grainy black-and-white photos showing the agony of Clarke. As

Australia's team doctor, I had rushed to his side and pumped oxygen into his unconscious body. I cradled him in my arms trackside and wept with sheer frustration over the utter stupidity of the old men in suits who had reduced him to a wreck.

Journalist Alan Trengove, who was covering the Mexico City Olympics for the *Melbourne Sun* newspaper, described my embrace of the great runner as one of the most definitive moments in the history of Australian sport.

It was most certainly one of the most definitive in the 'Life of Brian'.

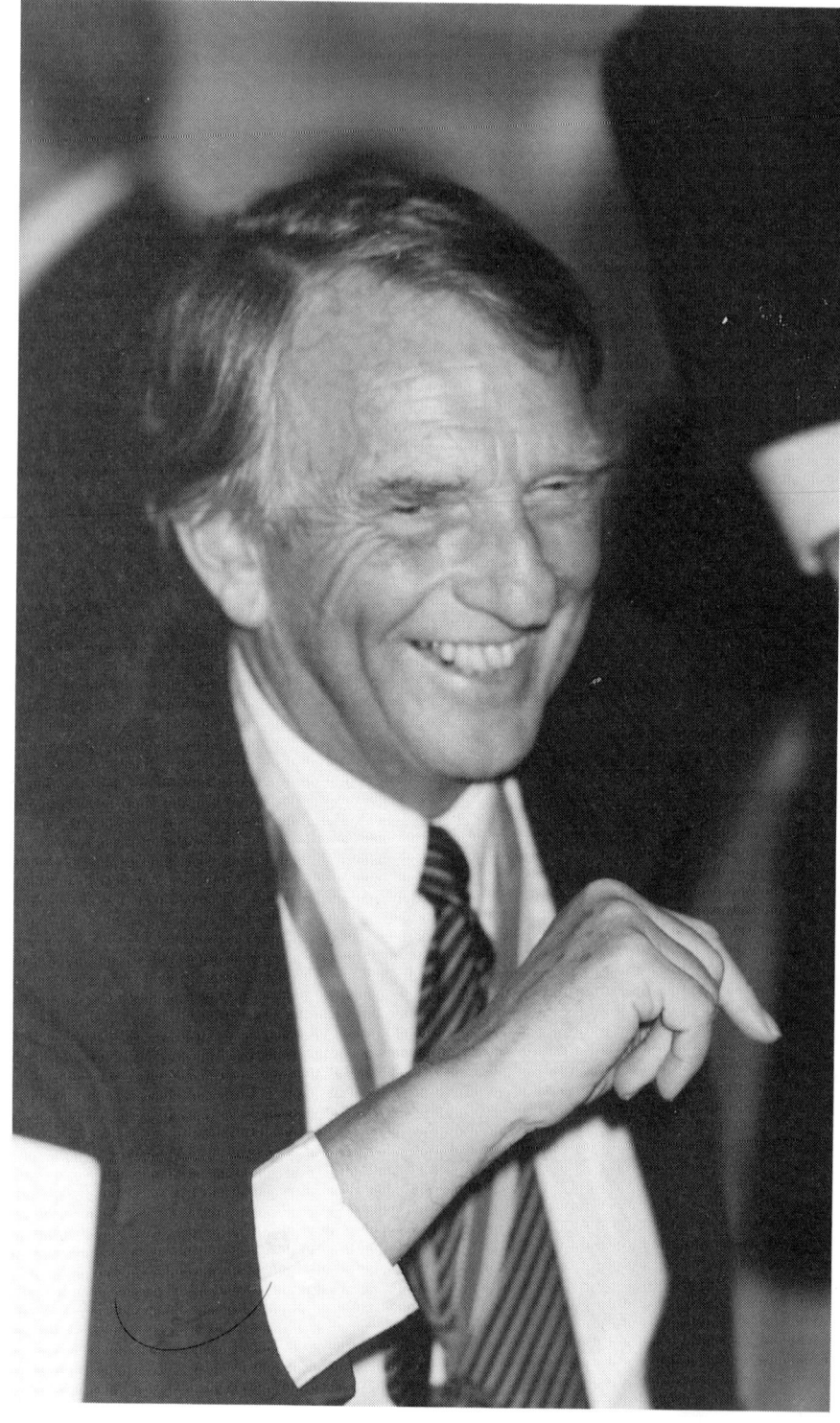

When I left school, I had absolutely no idea what I wanted to do. If truth be known — probably nothing.

1. THE KID FROM GLEBE

'YOU SHOULD WRITE your memoirs, Doc.' I'm not sure how often I heard those words. But I heard it again from one of my old mates at a reunion one day when a few of us were sitting around yarning about old times and the often very funny characters and sporting heroes we've met or worked with over the years.

While not too sure who broached the subject that day, I certainly remember my reply, 'I have no intention of writing any memoirs. If there is one thing I cannot stand it's a book that starts off saying something along the lines of ... I was born at an early age ... my father hated me and was mean to me ... and we had no money ... and had to walk to school in the snow without shoes ... that sort of thing. Even if it were true, you would be spared that.'

However, they persuaded me to put down on paper some of the yarns I've recounted over the years. And thanks to the persistence of my publisher I have reluctantly included a brief explanation of what turned a kid who loved sport into a doctor who pursued a career in sports medicine and ended up treating many of Australia's greatest cricketers, footballers and Olympic athletes, while watching — sometimes at disturbingly close quarters — the antics of coaches, managers and various, rather unconventional, journalists.

The inner Sydney suburb of Glebe, where I was born on Australia Day 1929, was not the trendy place it is today. It used to be a working class suburb known as the breeding ground for such diverse figures as

Frank Burge, a Rugby League pioneer who was tough enough to play first-grade as a 15-year-old schoolboy, and Edmund Barton, Australia's first Prime Minister and later the first Chief Justice of the High Court.

During the Depression, the government handed out coupons to the most needy people. These coupons were swapped for groceries. The government reimbursed my father in exchange for the coupons. This was how he was paid for most of the groceries he sold.

I was very conscious that many kids in Glebe had to go to school without shoes or a coat in the winter and some of my friends, often quite bright, had to leave school at the age of about 13 because they couldn't afford to stay on. This certainly helped shape my moral and political attitudes that I have carried into adult life.

I can't say it was fun, but it certainly wasn't an awful childhood. School teachers and my father were not averse to handing out a whack, but I can only remember being really belted once. That was for something I didn't do, so that hurt. All the other times I would have deserved it, I suppose.

I was named Alfred after my dad, but for some reason was always addressed by my second name, Brian. I always preferred Brian — never really liked Alf. And *The Life of Alf* doesn't really have a ring to it.

I really loved my mother, Dorothy. She was a very intelligent woman who had studied to be a schoolteacher. One of her colleagues at Teachers College was Bill O'Reilly, later to become one of Australia's greatest cricketers ('He was a nice boy, but drank a bit too much,' she said about the man the cricketers dubbed 'Tiger'). It was through her efforts that I ended up studying for the last three years of high school at Sydney's famous — but down-to-earth — GPS school, St Joseph's College in Hunters Hill.

Dorothy Corrigan certainly excelled as a mum to my two sisters, Berenice and Christine, and myself but died far too early from cancer, passing away on the first day of my final medical exams. I did not think I could continue with them, but before she died she had made me promise I would do them. It was very hard.

I'M NOT REALLY sure why I ended up as a doctor. I could say that I wanted to devote my whole life to helping ease the suffering of humanity, but that would be complete bullshit. When I left school, I had absolutely no idea what I wanted to do. If the truth be known — probably nothing. There were some chemists in the family and my father thought that pharmacy would be a good profession for me and started to steer me in that direction.

I received very high marks in the Leaving Certificate (the forerunner of today's Higher School Certificate) and obtained a scholarship to university. My mother actually decided my future for me. She reckoned I wanted to be a doctor and enrolled me in the medical faculty at Sydney University. At first, I hated it like mad. I wasn't terribly interested in first year subjects such as Botany and Zoology, which were compulsory probably because professors in these subjects were keen to keep a job for themselves and persuaded the powers-that-be that the study of plants and animals would help blokes like me become better doctors. The system now is completely changed and medical students are introduced to clinical medicine from the start. In my case, there was also the fact that I really didn't bother to study much, just scraping through exams until I got to my fourth year and the practical side in the hospital. Then it all sort of clicked into place and, from then on, I loved every minute of it.

My other love has always been sport. Since a boy I was always fascinated by the statistics of sports. How fast people ran or how high or far they jumped, the averages of cricket's batsmen and bowlers ... all that Trivial Pursuit sort of thing. Over the years, I have played many different sports — most of them poorly, all of them enthusiastically. My truly great passion has always been cricket, which I played in the lower grades until I was 36 years old. I have always enjoyed training and strive, even all these years later, to keep fit.

THERE WAS A Joey's 'younger set' which I joined soon after leaving school. It was great fun, picnics, parties, and so on — one sad thing about the youth of today is that there are no such organisations where kids can meet that is not a pub. There was a group of about 40 boys and 40 girls who soon paired off, as these things inevitably happen. We all have remained great friends ever since. Except for one small detail — there are now only four of the boys left, all the others having died. There was one particular guy there that had his eye firmly fixed on one of the girls, Monica. She asked me for my protection from him. She obviously

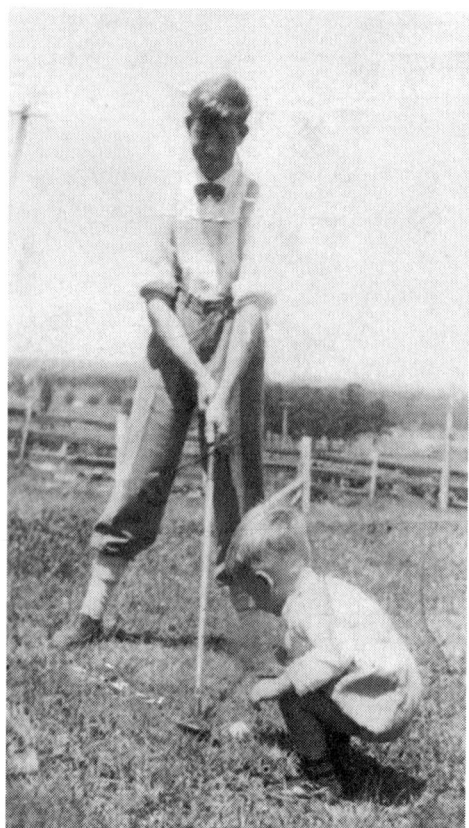
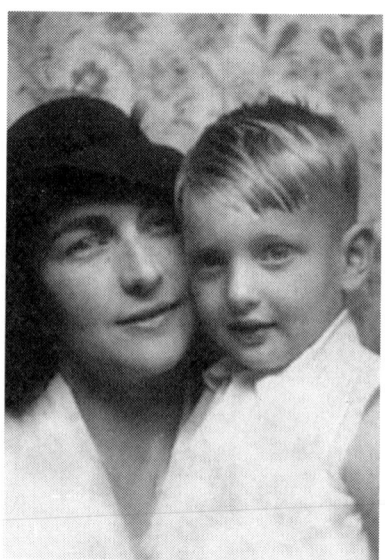

(LEFT) My sporting life started early. Learning to duck as my father tees up. (ABOVE) With my mother, Dorothy. (BELOW) My wedding to Monica. The best man, Jim Dixon, is behind in the second row.

(ALL BRIAN CORRIGAN'S COLLECTION)

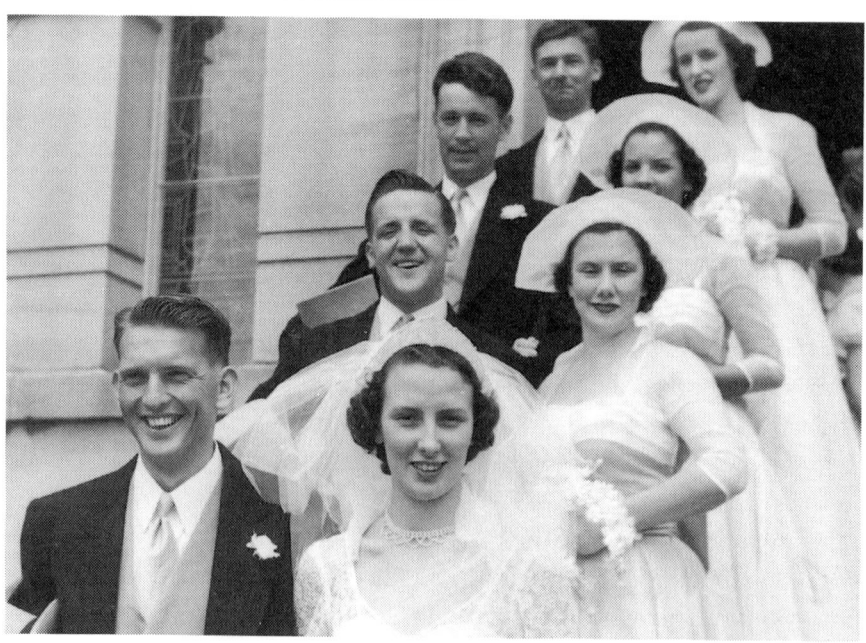

recognised my great potential and whisked me off. In all truth I have never regretted it.

And we are still together. Monica and I were married at the end of my university studies. There can be no doubt at all about the strength and support Monica has given me over so many decades. We have five kids, Sue Ellen, Carolyn, Shayne, Joanne and Dominic, and I love them so much. They are great and normal kids, get on well together, are solid citizens and great role models for our 14 grandchildren. That is a huge achievement. But it is all due to Monica. I could not have accomplished anything without her. I was away a lot with my work and she had the job of looking after all the kids and did that to perfection. I owe her an immeasurable debt.

SP OR NOT SP!

I needn't explain that Australians are notorious gamblers. When I was a kid in the days before the TAB was in operation, most suburbs had their local illegal SP (starting price bookie). In Glebe, the SP man was an important local dignitary who ran his betting establishment in the basement of the Town Hall. The boy who lived next door and I had a job of a Saturday afternoon working as a cockatoos, meaning we were supposed to watch for the approach of the police and warn the bookie about it. For this we were paid a shilling a day, a lot to us in those days. But we couldn't tell our parents about it. If we had done so we would probably have been skinned alive. Anyway, we never ever saw any police sneaking up on the premises and, as the glamour soon wore off, I became bored with standing around having nothing to do and quit.

In reality we were quite redundant. After all, the police used to have £10 (none of their own money having to change hands before the race, of course) on the winner of the last race. If it came in as a short-priced favourite, the bookie did not have that much to lose and could relax. But if it was a long shot, he still had to pay out on the odds and that could amount to a large sum. I didn't understand much about such things as corruption in those days, but the clandestine nature and the sneaking around left me with a distinct dislike for gambling — an aversion I still have today.

All this is to introduce a story about one day when I had just started at Joey's boarding school. I was standing in a long queue to buy some schoolbooks, when a boy I had never met before came up, said his name was Jim Dixon and asked if I would do him a favour.

'Oh, yes. But first, what is the favour?'

'Well, I'm carrying a lot of betting slips in my pocket. The headmaster has called me up to his office and I am afraid I will be caught with them, and you know what that means.'

'No, tell me.'

'I will be expelled, of course,' he explained.

'Well, you had better leave them with me.'

He went away with a most worried look on his face. Suddenly I thought to myself, 'This could be a very big mistake. What would my parents say if I were to be caught?'

Jim got back after 15 or 20 minutes, grinning broadly.

'How did you get on?' I asked.

'Great,' he beamed at me. 'The headmaster only wanted me to give him some tips for the races, because he is going there on Saturday. How did you get on?'

I thought this could be a good time to get even with him for causing me all that worry, so I replied, 'Not so good, mate. I'm in terrible trouble. I got caught with all the slips in my pocket.'

'Look, don't let that worry you. I'll make it up to you.'

'Oh, yeah! How will you do that?'

'You can be the best man at my wedding,' was his answer.

Twelve years later I was. And he was the best man at mine.

'She took me into her tiny office and opened a door into a smaller alcove. There was the embalmed body of a man, standing to attention in his World War I army uniform.'

2. A COUNTRY PRACTICE

MY MEDICAL LIFE began in the faraway 1950s as a GP in a small country town in the New England area of northern New South Wales. I have always been mindful about how much I learned about medicine and people as a country practitioner because you had to rely so much on your own judgment. After all, the base hospital was far away and transport wasn't as readily available back then as it is today.

The diminishing number of doctors willing to enter country practice is, or should be, a matter of grave concern to all Australians. As happens with so many facets of country life, no one seems to care sufficiently to do anything about it.

Country people have a wonderfully laconic way of dealing with their problems. Hence my own personal portfolio of unusual and intriguing stories from those early days in my medical career.

THE VERY FIRST patient I saw in my new practice was a pretty nineteen-year-old German girl working as an au pair. She told me she was worried about a rash. She was speaking in very broken English and I was uncertain as to what she was saying. I suggested it might be easier if we had a look at the rash. The surgery was quite large and had a separate examination room.

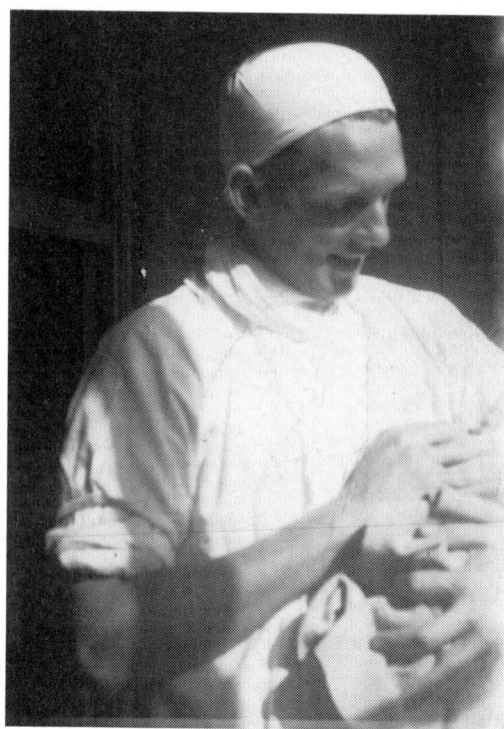

The first baby I ever delivered. Royal Hospital for Women, 1951
(BRIAN CORRIGAN'S COLLECTION)

When I went in to see her, she was sitting on the examination couch stark naked, except for a tiny towel. If I tell you I only looked at the rash, you will have to believe me. I told her to get dressed while I went back into the office to write out a prescription; handing it to her, I explained slowly that I would need to see her again to find out how she was getting on. She tossed her head and said something like 'Oh!' She grabbed the script, turned on her heel and walked out.

I was devastated, truly devastated. I was actually feeling quite sorry for myself. Here I was, first day in practice, she was my first patient, I had made a mess of it and I didn't really know why. I realised I had to get on with it. I composed myself as best I could and got ready for my second patient. As I walked out through the examination room, there was the young Fraulein, sitting up on the examination couch, once again naked.

I nodded my head.

'Thank you, miss. It's just what I had thought. You may get dressed now and leave.'

Ah, the trials of a young GP!

ONE OF THE hazards of country life was the every-present possibility of being bitten by a snake or a spider. One particular peril involved the ubiquitous redback spider that used to regularly inhabit outdoor toilets, where they could lurk under the seat, ready to dart out at unsuspecting victims as they were going about their business. The famous 'redback on the dunny seat'. They could inflict quite a nasty bite.

I received a call one day to tell me a redback bite victim was on his way to the surgery. When he arrived he was sitting in the back seat of the car, supported by two ladies. He was in agony — pale, cold, sweating, anxious and not saying a word.

'How are you, mate,' I asked while checking his pulse.

There was no answer. He just nodded his head.

'Where were you bitten?'

He sat up a bit and mumbled, 'Mate, if I had been one of these flamin' women, I would never have been bitten.'

Silly question.

ONE OF MY duties was to attend a clinic in a small nearby village. In the dim, distant past it had been a thriving mining town. But when the mine closed, the town slowly faded away. There had once been a doctor, but he, along with his daughter had committed suicide. Of course, being a small town there were plenty of nasty rumours about their deaths.

The town did have a cottage hospital but it was quite run down. Its matron, too, had seen better days. I wouldn't have been surprised had she been a nurse in the Crimea with Florence Nightingale.

We were walking around the grounds of the hospital one day when she noted, 'We've had a problem. A dead kangaroo was stuck down the well and we had a lot of trouble removing it.'

'Oh!' I mumbled, nodding my head. After we had walked a little further she exclaimed, 'There has been a terrible outbreak of diarrhoea among all the patients. Most of them are awfully ill.'

'Mmm. I wonder what caused that?' I replied, putting on my best consultant's voice.

'I've already told you,' she snapped in an exasperated tone as if she was scolding a little boy. 'We've had a dead kangaroo in the drinking well.'

On another occasion when we were walking around the hospital, she suddenly turned to me and asked, 'Would you like to meet my father?'

'Um … well … yes,' I said, perplexed as I was certain he could not still be alive, such was the matron's vintage. She took me into her tiny office and opened a door into a smaller alcove. There was the embalmed body of a man, standing to attention in his World War I army uniform, surrounded by personal memorabilia with a lamp burning beside him.

'Father, this is Doctor Corrigan,' the matron said. I wasn't sure what to say, but I think I mumbled something back to the cadaver.

It was a pretty spooky moment.

ONE OF MY patients was a hard-working grazier. And he had reaped the reward for his years of hard work. He was very, very rich. The locals called him 'Hurricane', as in hurricane lamp — he was a bit dim.

Many years later when I was in practice in Sydney, he came to see me about a very painful right hip. I explained that what he needed was a then newly-developed operation, a total hip replacement. He seemed most impressed and asked who was the best surgeon in the world when it came to hip replacements. I thought that would be Professor Jack Charnley in Manchester, England, the man who had perfected the procedure.

'All right, Doc, can you get me an appointment with this Professor Charnley, in a hurry?'

I did. And Hurricane flew off to Manchester for the operation. Not a cheap excursion in those days. He returned from England as pleased as Punch with his new hip and promptly sent Charnley a most expensive present.

A year or so later Hurricane was in London and decided to give Charnley a ring to report his progress and explain how he intended to drive up to Manchester to have his hip checked out. He was certain the surgeon would see him … if only for the size of the present he had sent. Hurricane eventually managed to get through to the very busy Charnley, who asked how his hip was.

'Well, it's free of pain, but I just don't feel it is quite right.'

'There is no such thing as one of my hip operations being not quite right,' the great man said frostily as he banged the phone down in Hurricane's ear.

So much for being a multi-millionaire from the colonies.

THERE WERE TWO lovely old ladies, sisters who lived together. They were often seen, when shopping in the street, with a smile and kind word for everybody they met. I saw them in the surgery one day for some minor problem when they hinted to me about some dark family secret, but I thought such sweet ladies were probably being a bit melodramatic.

One of the ladies rang me one day, most distressed. I could hear screams in the background. Could I come to their house urgently to see their younger brother? I thought it quite strange that they had never mentioned a brother before. When I saw him, it was fairly obvious that the brother, who now had the DTs, had been a heavy drinker for some time.

'He has to be admitted to hospital, urgently,' I told them.

'Oh please, you mustn't do that,' one pleaded. 'We would never ever be able to get over the shame of it.' It turned out that the reason why no one had ever seen him around the town was he had never been allowed out of the house.

'Can't you just give him an injection,' was the tearful request.

'Well, OK, I'll try, but it's against my better judgment.'

Now, I don't know if you have ever tried to give someone an injection as he was crawling up the wall while being chased by demons, as you might imagine it is a difficult procedure. Luckily he was slightly built and I finally gained enough control to give him an injection in his buttock. He then started to settle down and finally went to sleep. Even more miraculously, after this he went cold turkey and never drank again.

The sisters were tremendously grateful, but I felt awful about it. Whenever I saw him in the street, he would be walking with a pronounced limp, dragging his left foot. The injection had damaged his sciatic nerve, permanently. He would grasp my hand and with tears in his eyes say how eternally grateful he was. It seemed he believed I had cured his alcoholism with my injection. Then one day, he called in to say he had found a job where he could sit down and was leaving his sisters' house, and limped out of the surgery.

A year or so after this, the two sisters were sitting opposite one another having breakfast. The same tea and toast and marmalade they had consumed each and every day for years. Suddenly one calmly said to the other, 'Look at this!' She took the bread knife and slit her own throat, leaving a large, jagged wound. She didn't die but there was blood everywhere. This time there could be no argument, they had to get an ambulance and she was admitted urgently to hospital.

The two little old ladies became recluses after that and neither lived very long. No doubt the shame of it all killed them.

THEN THERE WAS the ex-serviceman. This patient was a big, well-built bloke … but a hopeless drunk. One day, he asked me to sign a travel form for him. Seems he had an eye injury which entitled him to travel to and from Sydney twice a year for a check-up. I felt sure he actually went to the big smoke to meet up with his old Army mates for a booze-up — and I was subsequently proved right. My belief that he was a no-hoper seemed to be confirmed when he said he couldn't and didn't work because of the psychological problems that he suffered after receiving his eye injury.

'How did you get that injury then?'

'Well, we were in the desert. I got a German bayonet through the eye.'

When I heard this I felt consumed with remorse. Here was I, who hadn't even been to a war, passing judgment on and doubting someone who had risked his life in battle, and had the scars to prove it. I felt I should never have doubted him. I reached for the form, ready to sign it, when I suddenly thought: 'Hang on! If you got a German bayonet through your eye, you'd be dead.'

'Yeah, doc, that's right.'

'Well, how did it really happen?'

'You see, I was in this brothel in Alexandria and I refused to pay the girl. She got so angry she stabbed me in the eye with a knitting needle. Don't tell anyone else though.'

'My lips are sealed. It's called the hypocritical oath.'

But I no longer felt any remorse.

'He hurled me across the room which was splattered with blood ... He was crawling towards me, mumbling, "Jack, I'm going to kill you".'

3. CITY LIMITS

AFTER RETURNING TO Sydney in 1956, I first worked at various locums before, later that year, settling down as a GP in a suburb on the northern beaches. I had gone there to help out a sick doctor in his practice at Dee Why, but his illness proved to be terminal. So I remained in the practice until 1961 when I went to England for further studies.

I soon found out that medicine and medical emergencies can be very different in the city. As people are pretty much the same wherever they may live, I found there were as many peculiar or unusual incidents in the city as out bush.

I think all male doctors could tell a story of harassment, to some degree or another, by a female patient. Most stories I've heard about follow a similar sort of pattern. Psychiatrists seem to be particularly vulnerable. One told me once that a female patient whom he had rebuffed sent him a present, a small cylindrical clinical torch to be kept in his top pocket. He showed it to me; it looked surprisingly like a penis. But the light would never flash.

One of the cases etched in my memory involved a married couple. He was a mild-mannered civil servant. She had probably once been quite a beauty, but her looks were rapidly fading. For the sake of confidentiality, I'll call them Mr and Mrs Thomas. I used to see them now and again for a variety of minor problems. One day she came in to say her husband had given her an expensive present for her birthday —

a series of allergy injections. What a bizarre thing to do, I thought, particularly as I had never previously seen her for any allergy problems. I felt compelled to ask a few questions.

'Why would you want a series of injections as a present?'

'Because every night I dream about you, and you are sticking this long thing into me.'

'Mrs Thomas, I won't be seeing you any more, you can see one of the other doctors if you like for your allergy treatment.'

A SOMEWHAT DIFFERENT scenario occurred when I had earlier done a locum in a two-man practice, filling in for one of the doctors who had suddenly taken ill. The remaining doctor was very tall, very handsome and very attracted to the ladies, and vice versa. He was busy one day and asked me to do a house call for him. A lady had rung to say she had injured her back and couldn't move.

I knocked on the door and the voice inside called out the standard, 'Who's that?'

And the standard reply, 'It's the doctor.'

As the door opened I caught a flash of black frilly underwear and lots of bare flesh.

'Where's the proper doctor, then?'

'He won't able to get here today.'

'Oh, you'll have to wait outside until I get dressed.'

She quickly twisted around and just as quickly disappeared.

'There's not too much wrong with your back, madam,' I decided.

BOXING IS A brutal game, one that attempts to glorify itself with grandiose titles such as the noble art of self-defence. It is never noble but cruel and vicious and its main object is to punch someone about the head until he is knocked out or their brain is sufficiently scrambled that they can end up becoming punch-drunk or develop Parkinson's disease, as with Mohammad Ali.

There may be an art to boxing, but I have always found it extraordinary that boxers are not allowed to hit below the belt, lest the opponent injures their testes, yet they are allowed to inflict damage to the infinitely more important membranes around the brain. Surely the penalty should apply so that you preserve the brain and not the balls, and points be awarded for that skill?

Have you ever knocked anyone out? Or thought about it? Or thought how you would go about it? I most certainly hadn't until the night I received a call to a less salubrious part of town from a sobbing, distraught woman, whom I had not previously met. I knocked on the door. It was opened by a fairly big man, unsteady, obviously very drunk, completely naked and covered with blood. That was about all I had time to observe before he grabbed me by the throat, yelling, 'Jesus, Jack, I've been looking for you.'

With that, he hurled me across the room which was splattered with blood. Shaken, I got to my feet and turned to face him. He was now on his hands and knees, he might have slipped because of the grog or from the blood on the floor. He was crawling towards me mumbling, 'Jack, I'm going to kill you.'

Friendly! What do you do? I thought about trying to get away, but that wasn't possible. I realised I was going to have to knock him out. How do you do that? In the movies it looks so easy, you just clench your fists and bang someone about the head and continue punching away for some minutes, without ever seemingly doing any damage to the hands. I was most conscious that my clenched fist striking against any man's head would be much more likely to break the bone in my knuckle than to damage him. So, just as he reached me, still on his hands and knees, I clasped my two hands together and swung them around to hit him with a chopping-like action with the side of my hand. It was a pretty solid whack. Whether it was because of that or because he was so drunk I don't know, he fell flat on the floor at my feet.

I found a terrified wife and two children, bashed and bleeding profusely, trying to hide in the bedroom, and said, 'You'd better get out of here quick, you haven't got much time.'

The back door was locked — he had taken the key — and the family were so petrified they refused to go through the lounge where he was lying out cold. The four of us had to scramble out through a window to get to my car. The still-crying lady had a relative living nearby and I rang the police from there, told them what had happened, and asked them to come quickly. They did. The woman told me he was only aggressive when he was drunk. On this night he had got really drunk and wanted to kill his wife and kids and himself. I met the police outside the front of the house. They went through the blood-spattered front room and found him in the bedroom, still crawling on his hands and knees.

He looked up at me and said, 'I remember you, Jack.'

Before he could utter another word, the policeman gave him the most God-Almighty thump across the head with some sort of truncheon. It really was a knockout.

The postscript to this story … a few weeks later, Monica, the kids and I went away on a holiday and my brother and sister-in-law, Bill and Noelene, came to mind the house for us. There was a knock on the door one night and a wild-looking man was standing there with an axe in his hand.

'I'm looking for Jack, this is where he lives.'

He was assured there never had been any Jack living there, and thankfully after a time he went away, mumbling to himself. Our terrified in-laws never came to mind the house again.

I still don't know who the real Jack was.

THEN THERE WAS the case of the inheritance. One day in 1960 a pleasant, middle-aged man turned up at the surgery, introduced himself and explained he hadn't come for himself but had a special request. He wanted me to keep his old mother alive. It turned out that she had Alzheimer's disease. I explained that there was no cure, although I was sure he knew that already. He agreed there was no cure, but he just wanted me to keep her alive. She could have any treatment I thought might help.

When I went to see her, I realised that her illness was very well advanced, and had been for years. I again explained to her son that I couldn't cure her but he insisted that I just needed to keep her alive. One of the major problems was that his mother spent most nights roaming the streets and was a menace to traffic. The police were getting most irate at having to take her home all the time. She obviously needed to be in a nursing home but the son was insistent, 'No way! Mother must never be put in a home. I am absolutely adamant about that.'

'Then she has to have a nurse at home who can look after her 24 hours a day,' I replied. 'And that could be a bit expensive.'

'I think I know of one,' he said. 'I think she would be very good for the job, I'll hire her. Money is no object.' (I am always suspicious when I hear that. It usually means that they have no intention of paying anyone. But for some reason I did trust this man).

My heart sank when I first met the nurse he had hired. She was an old lady, whose nursing training had probably consisted of a few days as a receptionist in a private hospital somewhere. Her new employer thought the world of her.

I got to know the son fairly well after a while and said I thought there had to be more to the story than mere filial devotion. He invited me home where he showed me a large room stacked with law books and old charts. He said he did not work any more but had studied for a law degree, which he had recently attained. Then he told me his story.

Back in 1795, his forebears, for services rendered to Governor Hunter, had been granted a huge tract of land beside a lake and it was to be kept by them and their descendants in perpetuity. It was now worth a very considerable fortune.

However, the State government was now disputing the land title and was trying to dispossess the family. The son had fought long and hard in the Courts, but had lost in all of them. It had been decreed that the family's title would last until his mother died, after which the Government would resume all the land. That is why he had decided to study law to fight the case himself. His last resort was appealing to the Privy Council in England (back in the 1960s it was still possible) and he was busy preparing the brief.

He said he was absolutely certain he could win his case, but it was essential his mother remained alive. If she died his case would be null and void (notice how lawyers love using tautologies, there is a long list of them. They are probably paid by the word). So would I keep visiting her and the 'nurse' every week to check on her?

When I next went to visit them, this elderly nurse reported that the mother's nocturnal rambles were getting worse and she was exhausted trying to keep up with her. She asked if the mother could have some sort of sleeping tablet? I wrote the script with strict instructions that only one was to be administered each night. Luckily, that tablet seemed to be some help, at least for a while.

Some time later the 'nurse' rang me. In a very reasonable tone of voice, she asked, 'You know those tablets you gave me? Could I give her two at a time?'

'Oh, I suppose that would be all right, if you had to.'
'What about six at a time?'
'No, most definitely not.'

Still in the same reasonable tone, 'then could you come around as quick as you can? She looks a bit blue.'

A bit blue? When I got there, the mother had been dead for several hours. I called the police as I thought they may want to make it a coroner's case, but they said definitely not, to let things be. Fair enough. After all I did not really know for sure if the tablets had killed her.

The son took her death with surprising calm. I felt he had been expecting it. I never had the heart to tell him exactly what happened that night.

And to complete the story … yes, the government did resume all the land and all that is left of the government grant is a suburb named after him.

IN THE OLD days on the northern beaches, I had one minor obsession — always trying to park my car in the main street right outside my surgery, where it would sit, free of charge, all day. Each day it was a bit of a challenge to find how close to the surgery I could park. I only mention all this because no one could possibly do that nowadays. Even if you could find the space, the streets are littered with parking meters which allow you to remain there only at considerable expense for just half an hour.

At one time, I had a brand new Holden. I parked it across the road and periodically would glance at it from the surgery. One afternoon, a big man in shirtsleeves and braces crossed the street, put a key in the car door, got in and started to drive it away. What the hell? I bolted through the front door of the surgery to see my car waiting to turn right at the next corner. A taxi was parked outside, so I jumped into the front seat, yelling dramatically, the immortal words from the movies: 'Follow that car!' There was one slight problem, however. The cab had two old ladies in the back and they were just saying to him, 'We would like to go to Manly, please, driver.' The taxi driver, I was quick to pick up, was a man of very nasty temperament. He started to abuse me telling me, in words he should never have used in front of those dear old ladies, to get out of his cab.

'Look,' I said, watching the rapidly receding rear of my Holden. 'That's my car and it is just being stolen.'

Never have you seen such a transformation. My now genial taxi driver noted, 'If there is one thing I cannot stand, it's some bastard … sorry ladies … who steals a car. Don't worry, mate, I'll get it back for you. Hang on!' With that, we took off down the main street, and we did literally have to hang on. He grabbed his radio and called base to report what was happening. As luck would have it, I recognised the voice on the other end as that of a friend, Steve Hawthorn.

'Is that you, Steve?'

'Yeah, Doc. Don't worry, we'll get it back for you. One thing we can't stand is some bastard who steals a motor car.'

He got on his blower to call the police and all available cabs in the area to come urgently. The driver was reporting back which streets my car was turning into. The two old ladies in the back were saying, 'Are you sure this is the way to Manly?'

Finally, we saw the car in front of us as it pulled into a quiet street and parked. The driver started to get out just as we screeched to a halt behind it. My cabbie with his re-discovered nasty temperament jumped out, headed straight for the driver and started to abuse the very startled man. I was not in such a hurry, for two reasons. The first, as already mentioned, was that he was a very big man, bigger than both of us, and the second was that the braces he was wearing had 'police issue' stamped on the buckle.

By this time the street was starting to fill up from all directions with taxi cabs, one driven by Steve Hawthorn, and a police car with its siren screaming. The big man was explaining to the excited throng (all the neighbours had come out to witness the commotion) that he was a police officer and he had just bought a new Holden, the one here was definitely his. To prove it, we should all look at the number plate.

We did just that and it was mine. As things started to settle down, the big man apologised profusely and offered to drive me back to the main road to sort it out. I went over to say sorry to the two old ladies for the inconvenience caused. They told me not to worry as they had not had so much fun for ages and they loved the police sirens. I thanked the cab driver who would take no payment for all his trouble.

'Happy to help, mate,' he said as he headed off towards Manly at last with the two old ladies.

The big man drove me back to the surgery. We parked in the same spot as before … right behind an identical Holden. The same key fitted both locks. He said sorry, he did take the wrong car. I said not to worry, simple mistake, and we shook hands.

That afternoon, I had a visit from a policeman who took out his notebook and said he believed I had reported a stolen car. I told him that I wasn't the one who reported it stolen. Steve was. I also pointed out the problem had all been sorted.

The policeman was insistent. The police force took it very seriously, because one thing they couldn't stand was some bastard who steals motor cars. He had to report the details. Did I want to lay any charges?

'Not at all … anyway, he was a sergeant of police.'

'Oh, was he? Well, we needn't worry then.' He hurriedly put the notebook back into his top pocket, turned on his heel and walked out.

THERE WAS A young football player whose main attributes were that he had a perfect build and trained as hard as anyone I ever knew. His great ambition was to play for Australia, but his prospects of that were quite limited because of one small problem — he didn't have sufficient talent. He was good but only half as good as he thought he was.

One day while playing he twisted and fell, injuring his lower rib cartilage. Anyone who has had such an injury can testify that it is extremely painful for such a small injury. And it takes ages to heal. I told him this and said there was no active treatment for it. I'm not too sure how he took that, but about a week later there was a photo of him in the local paper, sitting up in a hospital bed, pyjama top off, showing off his very good physique and surrounded by seemingly adoring nurses. I felt bad because it seemed I had missed some diagnosis. I called into the hospital. He explained how he would be in hospital for a while because no one could diagnose the problem. I felt reassured when I found his rib injury was still the problem and there were no other complications. As I left he asked me if I would get him a magazine he wanted to read. He was in hospital for another week.

A week after his discharge from hospital, his mother rang me at the surgery, crying, to tell me that Miles had been urgently admitted to a different hospital because he had suddenly lost his memory. I drove there as fast as I could, again feeling awful that I had missed something.

Same thing! There he was sitting up in bed, now surrounded by anxious relatives, most of them crying. They confirmed his problem was this memory loss and he was to undergo a series of nasty tests.

Just as I was leaving, he sat up in bed, and said, 'Hey, Doc, I still have that magazine you lent me, I'll get it back to you as soon as I can.'

As I left I was able to assure his mother that his memory would improve very quickly. He was discharged the next day.

'Pretend you're in a swimming pool and a hungry shark is coming for you.'

4. COTTON'S FIELD

AS A MEDICAL student at Sydney University, I had come directly in contact with Professor Frank Cotton, the professor of physiology. He had formed a group consisting mainly of students that became known as the 'guinea pigs'. Professor Cotton was dubbed 'The Father of Sports Science' by the future Olympic swimming coach Forbes Carlile. After all the Professor was the first person in Australia to take any interest in what we now know as sports medicine — although it was pretty basic stuff back then in the 1940s.

Cotton had been a top-class swimmer, who had narrowly missed out on selection in the 4 x 200-metre relay team for the 1924 Paris Olympics. It was a great disappointment for Cotton because he was originally in the side but lost his spot when officials ordered a second selection swim. The team, headed by swimming legend Boy Charlton, won a silver medal.

The Professor was an interesting character, often regarded as eccentric, a real boffin. He worked out of a small, rudimentary laboratory, with very basic equipment.

But in so many respects Frank Cotton was way before his time. He pioneered early attempts to introduce scientific methods into the pursuit of elite physical performances in sport, and especially in rowing and swimming. He also tried to devise methods to test fitness. Sadly, he was often perceived as doing little more than taking someone's pulse. And he had some rathe weird ideas. I remember him one day asking me to increase my pulse rate.

'How can I do that?' I asked innocently.

'Pretend you're in a swimming pool and a hungry shark is coming for you,' he suggested. Come again!

There was another incident I clearly recall. Cotton handed me a text book and noted, 'There are a lot of mistakes in this book. Find out what they are. That's the way you'll learn what's right.'

I often wonder what would have happened if I didn't find the mistakes.

Forbes Carlile was a lecturer in physiology at the same time Cotton was at the university. Forbes has the distinction of being, in 1952, Australia's first Olympic representative in modern pentathlon — a gruelling event involving horse riding, swimming, athletics, shooting and fencing. Although heavily involved in coaching some of Australia's Olympic swimming hopefuls for the 1952 Helsinki Olympics, he was given permission to take time off and compete in the pentathlon there, in which he finished a creditable twenty-fifth out of a field of 51. He had also once taken part in a marathon, where he ran in searing heat, collapsed and ended up near death in hospital with kidney failure. I often got the impression that the marathon run was just another experiment to Forbes.

Cotton and Carlile were approached by Australian swimming chiefs after a relatively disappointing display by the Aussies at Helsinki. The authorities were worried that the home side at the 1956 Melbourne Olympics would be an embarrassment in the eyes the world. Thanks to these two scientists that never happened. In some cases they switched distance swimmers to the sprint events and vice versa — with outstanding results. The most notable was Jon Henricks, who when switched to the sprints won two gold medals.

It is now history how Australia dominated the pool at Melbourne. Sadly, Frank died in 1955 a year before the Melbourne Games without enjoying his success. But he had sown a seed in me that led to my subsequent interest in sports medicine.

THE SPECIALTY OF sports medicine, linking my two great loves, did not exist in Australia when I first started out as a young doctor in 1953. It had a long tradition in Europe, but did not commence here until the 1956 Melbourne Olympics, at which time the International Olympic

Committee (IOC) insisted such an organisation be formed. It was the forerunner of the Australian Sports Medicine Federation but based then only in the Victorian capital.

A small band of the enthusiasts including Les Cotton, nephew of Frank and a real chip off the old block, and myself started a sports medicine group in Sydney in 1957. It was later to join with the Melbourne organisation. Little did I know at the time what an enormous impact this would have on my life. Back then, however, we simply realised that doctors would eventually have to go overseas and study sports medicine, and I planned accordingly.

While I was at university I had vague notions of becoming a psychiatrist and, indeed, had been offered a scholarship to study psychiatry at a major hospital on the shores of one of North America's Great Lakes. But I would have had to pay my own fare (as well as that of my new bride and our first daughter, Sue Ellen). As a young doctor this was completely out of the question.

My practice grew quickly and I soon had two more young colleagues with me. Each of us wanted to study overseas — so we agreed that when one went, the other two would help finance his travels from the practice.

I planned my visit to England to coincide with the 1961 Ashes cricket tour of the team led by Richie Benaud. By that time I had become quite involved with the NSW Sheffield Shield players in Sydney. This all came about by sheer luck. I had returned to my old country practice for a reunion one weekend in 1957. The visit coincided with a country cricket final. I was there watching the game. It was very hot and I was dressed only in a pair of shorts and sandals. The NSW Sheffield Shield selectors were there, too, and I was asked if I could give them a lift back to their hotel. They were quite surprised when I told them I was studying to be a sports medicine specialist as I hardly looked the part in my casual gear. But I got on well with them and they invited me along to a Sheffield Shield match in Sydney the following week. I wore a jacket and tie this time.

The selectors eventually asked if I could do something about the fitness of the NSW players. That's how my involvement with cricket at an elite level began.

I remember one of my first tasks was to help big fast bowler Gordon Rorke. He was a terrifyingly quick bowler, but his fitness was problematical.

You have to remember that few cricketers trained much in those days. Gordon also got little help at the nets because all the batsmen refused to face him because of his incredible speed.

Les Cotton and I took Gordon under our wing to help him build up his fitness. It paid off handsomely with his selection in the Test team to play England that season (1958–59). Sadly, we never got the chance to see the best of Gordon at Test level after that because in 1959 he contracted hepatitis in India, which left him desperately ill — a haggard collection of skin and bone when he arrived home. It brought his international career to a premature end after just four Tests (two each against England and India, with a bowling best of 3–23 against England and 2–30 against India).

SECOND OPINION

ALAN JONES

The top-rating Sydney breakfast radio personality for the past two decades. He moved to radio after success as a teacher and speech-writer for Prime Minister Malcolm Fraser. He was also a Rugby coach whose greatest contribution was steering the Australian Wallabies to victory against all four Home Nations on their 1984 tour of Britain and Ireland.

LARGER THAN LIFE

IT'S ALL SO long ago, but when I was teaching at The King's School in Sydney during the mid-1970s, Brian Corrigan was a pre-eminent figure in sports medicine in this country and, perhaps, in the world. We all remembered his dramatic attempts to breathe life into Ron Clarke in Mexico City. I shall never forget those images. It was an embodiment of the sensitivity of the man that Corrigan was in tears as Clarke was gasping for breath. As always, Corrigan prevailed.

Somehow or other, I was able to make contact with him and he was of inestimable value to my Rugby side as we tried to win a Premiership for the first time at The King's School in almost 40 years.

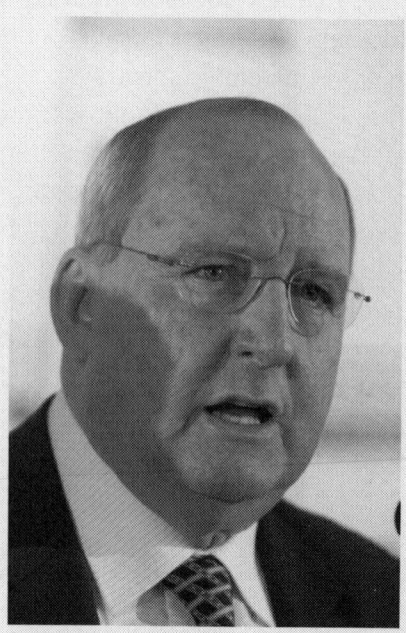

(AAP IMAGE/DEAN LEWINS)

Brian Corrigan was in the vanguard of sports medicine. It was unthinkable, at that time, for footballers to be going to someone like Brian Corrigan. That was minority behaviour. I remember him draining the bursa from the back of footballers' knees and he somehow got people on the paddock who, a week earlier, had been utterly immobilised. At the same time, I was coaching a squad of magnificent schoolboy athletes who were winning Australian titles. The comfort that I derived from knowing that I could pick up the phone any hour of the night or day and talk to Brian Corrigan was incalculable. He always delivered. His time and the inconvenience were never issues.

He's just a champion Australian.

And then, I was bold enough to presume upon him for my own problems. Painful back troubles. The response was the same. He gave me his every attention. Somewhere along the line he referred me to a variety of people. I somehow managed recovery from being a cripple who couldn't move, couldn't bend, couldn't stand up, thanks to Brian's contacts. Here I am today as if I never had the problem in the first place.

Brian revolutionised sports medicine. Early in his career he worked with one of the pioneers, Professor Frank Cotton. He did much more than Cotton. But he had an accessibility; a capacity to articulate the complicated medical background to a problem which the athlete could understand. That, in many ways, popularised the use of sports medicine. People didn't feel inhibited or intimidated when they were in the presence of Dr Corrigan.

Then, of course, there was the war against drugs. Well, he would salivate. He was a leader. He didn't want people to succeed through the use of drugs. We looked up to him, we admired him. And basically we said: 'Well, if Dr Corrigan feels this way, we must too.'

It's a tragedy that the drug trade has overtaken sport as it has and the Corrigans of this world have become, on this issue, something of dinosaurs. That is a tragedy. The leadership was always there from Brian Corrigan. The followers, over time, have fallen by the wayside.

There was always the larrikin in him. He was larger than life. He never crowded you with intellectual snobbery. He never lauded his superior intellectual strengths over you. He liked to laugh and joke. And he revelled in other people's successes. He loved to see 'his player' go out onto the field ... someone who was broken down a week ago and then turned the game ... because while Brian was treating people, he was also motivating them and talking to them, showing an interest in them. And they knew he would follow them through.

In the manuscript of life, few names are written as large as that of Brian Corrigan.

'The club doctor would have afternoon tea with the directors. He would never deign to sit on the bench and actually treat the players.'

5. MAKING A REPUTATION

SERENDIPITY PLAYS A huge role in the lives of each and every one of us. It definitely has done so on many occasions in mine.

At Lord's cricket ground in the London suburb of St John's Wood one Saturday on the Australians' 1961 Ashes tour, I found myself sitting next to a charming Englishman. As one does at the cricket, we were soon making conversation. It was a warm day and after a while he asked if I would like a beer. Did Freddy Trueman enjoy sledging Australian batsmen? There was no need to ask me twice. The Englishman enquired as to what I was doing in England. So I went through it all and told him how I was hoping to find a position at a London teaching hospital. Back then such a job was extraordinarily difficult to come by, and it was often unpaid. It is still the case today. My new-found friend smiled and said, 'Why don't you come and see me on Monday morning?'

'Oh, yes,' I replied. 'And where might that be?'

As it turned out, he was Professor Hugh Burt, who ran a large physical medicine department at London's University College Hospital (UCH). When I turned up on Monday morning, he offered me a position with his department. Best of all, it came with a salary!

My new job allowed me to study for degrees in physical medicine and rheumatology in both England and Scotland. I loved the job and enjoyed working with Professor Burt, for he was a great character. He

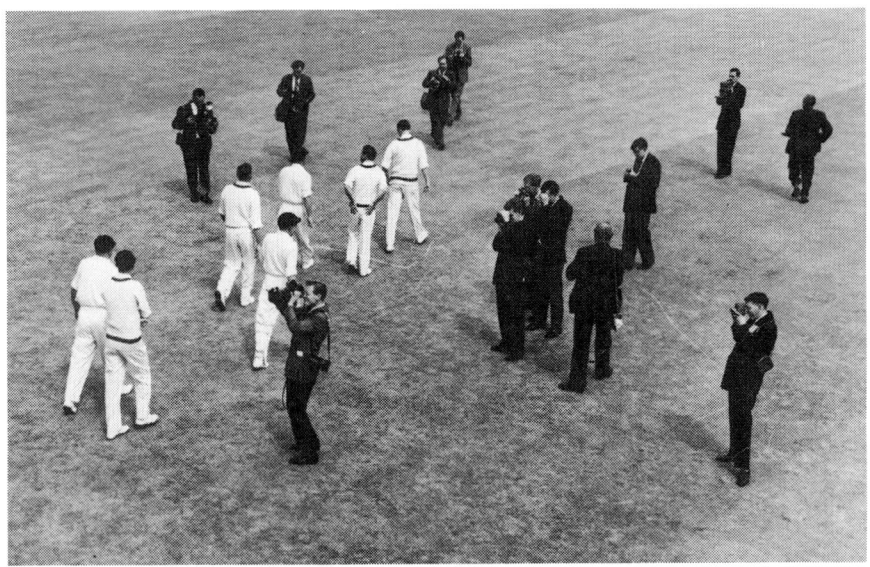

Richie Benaud's team walking on to the oval at Edgbaston, First Test, 1961. I am the guy with the camera, far right. (BRIAN CORRIGAN'S COLLECTION)

was always very busy and was often away at conferences. Every now and again, he'd be asked who did his work for him when he was away.

'Can't rightly say,' he would reply. 'I can only presume it is the same ones who do all the work when I am there.'

His ward rounds were eye-opening. He travelled at great speed through the wards, running up and down stairs, never using a lift, always surrounded by a large retinue of hospital registrars, physios, social workers, students and the invariable overseas heavy ... with me trying to keep up at the rear.

His other trick was that he would, at times, carry on at least two conversations at the one time. He was doing just that one day, when apropos of nothing he suddenly turned to me and said, 'Do you know, Corrigan, if you haven't made it by the time you are 40, you will never make it.' And with that, he turned to continue his conversation with the doctor on the other side about a patient who had a dreadful form of arthritis.

'What the hell is he talking about?' I thought to myself. I was about 30 years old at that time, and, not being too sure what he meant, I dismissed it. But when I reached 39, it suddenly came into my mind that I was shortly going to be 40 and I hadn't made it — whatever 'made it' meant. I became quite depressed and had a most miserable year until my 40th birthday. At that stage I suddenly decided: 'So what! I'm quite content with the way I am (or used to be, for that matter) and to hell with all that.' To this day, I do not know why he had inflicted that misery on me, for I am sure he never thought about that conversation again.

My message? Passing 40 is nothing special, as you do not reach your peak until at least 15 years after that.

ONE DAY AT the hospital I was being paged urgently. I mention this seemingly unimportant fact, because the paging system was in a most dilapidated condition. It rarely functioned at all, and was used sparingly.

I was being paged to go to Casualty. When I arrived I was told that an Irishman (why does it always have to be an Irishman?) had been admitted, and almost immediately had been pronounced dead. It turned out that he had started a new job that morning at Regent Park Zoo, just down the road. He had been given some sort of stick with a sharpened end and told that whenever he saw a piece of paper he was to pick it up. He came to a pit, saw a piece of paper and climbed over the fence to do as he had been told. The pit was a snake pit and he had been bitten by something venomous.

There was nothing I could do for the unfortunate victim, but I asked why the staff had paged me so urgently. They replied that as I was the only Australian in the hospital I would surely know how to treat snake bites. When I told them that the only time I had seen snakes was when I had taken my children to Regent Park Zoo, but they refused to believe me and asked if I could write the report about snake bites for the coroner. I did so, but only after finding some book in the hospital library about how to treat snake bites.

On another occasion, a Lascar seaman who spoke no English was admitted with severe heart failure. It was a baffling case as no one could work out the cause of the heart failure or why his condition was resistant to all treatment. One day, just before lunch, another sailor came up to me, pointed to the patient and mumbled, 'Him got beriberi.'

'OK, thanks,' I replied.

I went up to the lunch room, waited until there was a lull in the conversation, and casually announced, 'That seaman down in the medical ward, I think he has beriberi.'

Most of my colleagues looked at the Aussie upstart with grave scepticism, but the face of the senior physician suddenly lit up. He thumped the dining table and roared, 'My God, you're so right. What a clever diagnosis!'

Thus reputations are made.

WHILE IN LONDON in 1961, and again by sheer chance, I got a job as a doctor with the famous Arsenal Football Club.

Arsenal wasn't quite the dominant side it is today. At the time it was struggling under manager Billy Wright. Billy was one of the greatest players in the history of football. He had been capped 105 times for England, had been captain a record 90 times and also set a record of 70 successive international appearances.

Wright was short, standing just 172 centimetres, but was an incredible defender both on the ground and in the air. He was Footballer of the Year in 1952. Sadly, Billy didn't have the same success as a manager after he took over at Arsenal in 1962 and got shafted after four relatively unsuccessful years. His axing was unfair as he didn't have a lot to work with, but he knew how to pick talented youngsters, with nine of his signings forming the nucleus of the Arsenal squad that was to win the League and Cup double five years after his departure.

Billy was also a real celebrity … more so after marrying Joy, the eldest of the pop group the Beverley Sisters. Their wedding made headlines around the world. The football hero and the darling of pop music. The Beverley Sisters were bigger back then than the Spice Girls were at their peak. Teddie and Babs, the other two sisters in the group, were identical twins born on Joy's birthday. The group had hits on both sides of the Atlantic, including 'I Saw Mummy Kissing Santa Claus' and 'Drummer Boy'. And they regularly gave private concerts for the Royal Family at both Buckingham Palace and Windsor Castle. Posh and Becks (Posh Spice and David Beckham) — Joy and Billy were just as big as a celebrity couple in their era.

At Arsenal I joined the renowned sporting doctor Professor Alan Bass and respected physiotherapist Bertie Mee. The two of them helped change the way footballers were treated and subsequently played a major role in England's success in the 1966 World Cup.

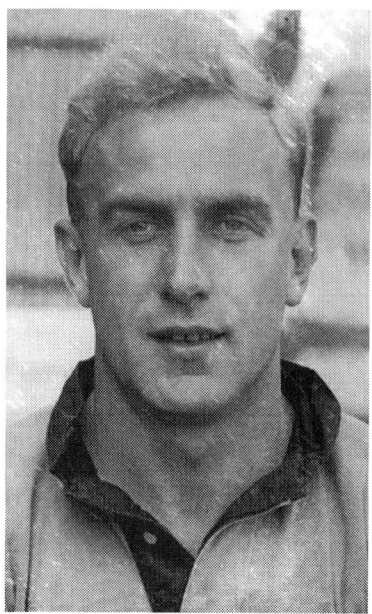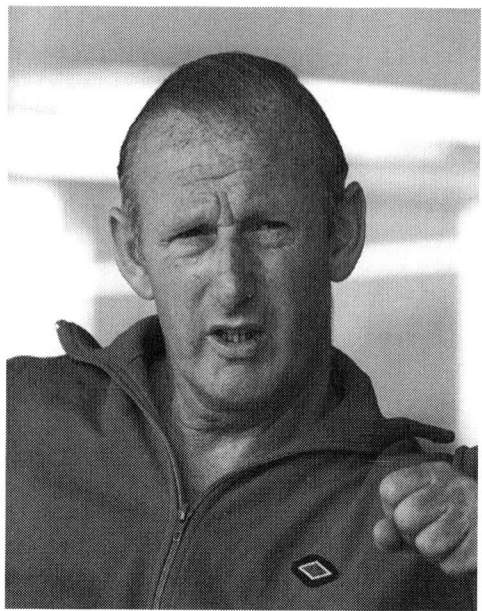

When I was the doctor at Arsenal in 1961, I worked with manager Billy Wright (LEFT), **one of the football greats, and physiotherapist Bertie Mee** (RIGHT), **who took over from Wright as manager.** (BOTH AAP IMAGE/PA SPORT)

Bass and Mee were the pioneers of a hands-on approach to sports medicine and the early treatment of sports injuries. Before their work at Arsenal the role of the football club doctor had been mainly a social one. The club doctor would sit up in the stand and have afternoon tea with the directors. He would never deign to sit on the bench and actually treat the players during a match, or after for that matter. Professor Bass and Bertie Mee changed all that — and I was lucky to be part of the team. I learned a great deal from them about training methods, diet and treatment of injuries.

Mee's efforts were rewarded when he was asked to take over from Wright as manager of Arsenal. The appointment shocked the football world, as Mee had never been a big name on the pitch. But he was a shrewd, proud man and no one's fool. With first-class player-management skills he became known for his ability to delegate tasks and motivate his players and steered Arsenal to the 1970–71 season double. Just as Alan helped change the role of the game's medicos, Bertie helped change how managers operated. Today's top managers owe a lot to the pioneering work of Bertie Mee.

> **SECOND OPINION**
>
> **ALAN DAVIDSON**
>
> One of the greatest all-rounders in the history of Test cricket. In 44 Tests he scored 1328 runs and took 186 wickets. He became a Test selector and president of the NSW Cricket Association for a record 33 years. Davidson was honoured with an MBE and an AM.

NEVER BEFORE, NEVER SINCE

IN THE 1960s, cricket tours were very different to those today. On an Ashes tour of England you would be away from your home and family for six or seven months. At times it could become quite harrowing. I missed my family terribly.

That's where Brian Corrigan came in. He worked as the team doctor, but he was much more than a mere medico. He was your family! Much of this had to do with his bewildering personality that boomed out at you ... his happy disposition ... the way he took the micky out of you, and accepted you taking the micky out of him.

He would invite you to his place in London.

'Mon will put a feed on and we'll have a chat,' Brian would explain. We'd sit out the back in that typical English garden. Daffodils, lupins, hollyhocks, snowdrops and whatever else in the corner. Just the right atmosphere to cheer up a lonely cricketer away from his family. These were truly precious moments.

Brian was more than a doctor. He was a confidant who understood how you were missing the folks back home. There was a certain closeness. This cricket tragic truly cared about his patients. It was more than just a great bedside manner. No matter how serious an injury, he would fight to keep your spirits up. They only give the famous 'baggy green' Australian cap to Test players, but if ever someone deserved recognition for his work in cricket it was Brian Corrigan. So when I retired I gave him my 'baggy green'. He has told me many times how much he treasures it.

IT WAS ON my first trip to England in 1953 that I was struck down by a crippling back problem. Then, during the 1961 tour, from the Second Test at Lord's on, I was a real mess. I used to sleep on the floor of my hotel room with a pillow under my stomach to keep my back off the ground. Brian knew the answer.

'I'm giving you three weeks off,' he said. 'Go down to UCH — the University College Hospital in London — and see Dr Alan Bass. He'll fix you up.'

All I knew was that Dr Bass was the club doctor for the famous Arsenal Football Club. But Brian's diagnosis was spot on — and the way to fix it was spot on, too. I'm not joking ... Dr Bass fixed me up in those three weeks, even though when I first went I couldn't even bend down to touch my knees. I was at the hospital each day and he put me through a series of exercises. He called it 'physiotherapy yoga'. Whatever the name, it worked. At first, all the exercises gave me excruciating pain as I exercised one leg at a time. Dr Bass, like Brian, had a soft, gentle manner ... a great connection with his patients. Within the allocated time I was able to easily bend down and put my hand flat on the ground. And in my first match back, against Ireland, I was racing around the boundary like a 16-year-old and hurling returns in over the stumps, not even stopping to take aim.

That was more than forty years ago. And whenever I feel the slightest twinge of pain in my back I return to the exercises prescribed by Dr Bass. I live by them.

LATE IN LIFE I became director of the Rothmans Sports Foundation and Brian was an immense help. During his career he had a hand in almost every sport played in Australia. And he changed those sports. Officials had usually been aloof and uncaring about the needs, medical and psychological, of the sportsmen and women under their control. If something was a success, the officials would take the credit. If something went wrong, they would blame the athletes.

Brian began to get players to understand their bodies and their limitations. And with his incredible record of successes he forced officials to realise that sports doctors were important. He got a real buzz out of that. The characteristic smirk on his face and the cackle that went with it reflected his pleasure.

I had never before seen such a person in the medical profession like Brian Corrigan. And I certainly haven't seen one since.

ONE OF THE most poignant moments of my life came in 1987 when I went to Government House in Sydney to receive an Order of Australia (AM) in appreciation of my services to cricket. By incredible coincidence Brian had been awarded an AM, too, and we were to receive our medals on the same day. It was in alphabetical order, so we were seated side by side.

In 2003, I was guest of honour at a lunch to thank me for my years in cricket. There were a few special people I wanted to be there: Bill Brown, my first captain; Richie Benaud, my Test captain in some of the glory days of Australian cricket; Stan Sismey and Tom Brooks from my early years in club cricket; and Brian. There were 740 people there on that day. But you couldn't miss the laughing face of the larrikin Brian Corrigan. He always stood out in a crowd!

'He remained so astonishingly unimpressed with himself.'

6. QUIETLY FLOWS THE DON

THANKS TO MY job as a sporting doctor I've been privileged to come in contact with some of those individuals lauded as sporting heroes and heroines. And it is interesting to note that in most cases in their day-to-day life they are just guys like you and me. They just have that extra talent that sets them apart in the sporting arena.

Sir Donald Bradman is undoubtedly Australia's greatest sports star. He is probably best remembered as 'Our Don Bradman' or, as befitted his iconic status 'The Don'.

We became good friends more than 40 years ago after our first meeting in 1957 while I was involved as doctor for the NSW cricket teams. On a couple of occasions he invited me down to Adelaide to visit him and his lovely wife, Jessie, who also became a firm friend, together with their daughter, Shirley. They formed such a brilliant partnership, Don and his childhood sweetheart, as devoted as any couple could ever possibly be. She was everything a wife could be to him, a veritable pillar for which he was eternally grateful. After she died, I rang to offer my condolences and he said that his life without her had become a nightmare.

One early visit was to consult with him about his neck pain, he had been given a diagnosis of fibrositis. There was a bit of a history to that particular diagnostic label. During the war, he first joined the RAAF in June 1940. Not many months later, he was transferred to the Army as a physical fitness instructor in Frankston. After about one year and several bouts of hospitalisation, he was invalided out with the diagnosis of fibrositis. It was a diagnosis as common in those days as rheumatism, both without any known underlying pathology. Soon after the war, a meeting of the British Orthopaedic Association announced that there was no such thing as fibrositis — it was all in the mind. (That august body was wrong in this pronouncement, as it was in so many others, but that is another story.) Some writers, such as Jack Fingleton, pounced upon this story, announcing that Bradman's illness was all in his mind, there was nothing wrong with him and he had shirked military service.

The problem was that Bradman's fibrositis was caused by an injury that had completely crushed a disc in his neck. This resulted in neck and arm pain caused by bony pressure on a nerve in his neck with weakness and wasting in his arm. At times he could not even lift his arm to shave. Treatments he had been having for his so-called fibrositis were making things worse. He was incredibly grateful to have all this sorted out and to have proper treatment.

Controversy dogged Bradman's whole life. Over the years, his relationship with many of his fellow cricketers was often as rocky as his home life was serene. These relationships can be divided by World War II.

Pre-war, the attitudes of a number of Australian cricketers towards him often ranged from dislike to disdain. After the War, again with a few exceptions, he had a new team of youngsters who looked up to him. Why this incredible difference?

I asked him about that one day over lunch. His explanation was jealousy. He said that life is like a tree. The bigger the tree grows the more people there are who can stand in its shade, and so there are more people to criticise, Bradman's explanation of what we know as 'the tall poppy syndrome'.

But I doubt that jealousy would be the whole story.

It has been said that when cricketers meet to recall all their funny stories, Bradman's name does not often come up. There may be many, many stories about him, but funny stories about him rarely exist, as befits what can be viewed as his ruthless approach to batting. He was also a non-smoker and a modest drinker ... most abstemious, preferring a cup of tea, never one to breast the bar and shout for the crowd, never the hail-fellow-well-met version of most cricketers. He was a man who often preferred his own company so that on tour he might spend time in his room listening to music and reading. He would say that after making a big score, he might be required to make another one the next day or so, and therefore needed the rest beforehand. In this, he might be contrasted with Brian Lara, who made two huge scores in a row from which, for one reason or another, he took a long time to recover before he could match these earlier run-scoring sprees, has said how much they had taken out of him. He probably could have done with the discipline that Bradman showed.

Bradman certainly did well to maintain his remarkable equilibrium amid all the constant adulation he received. This did not sit at all well with some team-mates who thought him distant, uncommunicative and aloof. Those were the days when fast bowlers, and even those slower, such as Bill O'Reilly, thought that at the end of the day, fluid replacement was mandatory. And fluid meant beer.

Bradman's team-mates certainly thought they had a few reasons to complain. When the boat carrying the Ashes-winning 1930 Australian team arrived in Australia from England, Bradman left it, travelling overland to capital cities, to be feted along the way by adoring crowds, leaving his team-mates to struggle back later. After his Test record score of 334 in Leeds in 1930, he received a telegram from soap magnate AE Whitelaw with a gift for £1000, more than double each player's tour allowance. He put it in his pocket and did not offer the other players so much as a drink and refused a request to shout them a meal.

A crowd of 40,000 at a Sheffield Shield game would vanish like a puff of smoke as soon as he got out, people would go back to work. It was not great encouragement for the batsman who followed, who might be someone of the calibre of Stan McCabe or Alan Kippax.

Some of his team members also had problems with his method of playing bodyline during the 1932–33 Ashes series. While most had to weather a severe battering from the hands of Douglas Jardine's array of fast bowlers, Bradman was determined, not unnaturally, not to be hit. He preferred, using his nimble footwork, to draw away to the leg-side and try to hit the ball to the unpatrolled off-side. He was hit once, but he said he saw no reason to become a martyr. Many did not agree with this method, some even expressed doubts about his intestinal fortitude.

During the bodyline series, the Australian captain, Bill Woodfull, after being hit under the heart, made his famous statement: 'There are two teams out there, one is playing cricket, the other is not. The game is too good to be spoilt. It was time some people got out of it.' His comments were made to the England team manager, Sir Pelham Warner, a member of the British Establishment and chairman of the MCC's selection committee.

Details of Woodfull's comments were leaked that night to renowned Australian sports writer Claude Corbett of the Sydney *Sun*. Who it was that leaked the story to Corbett has remained a mystery ever since. It had been assumed that only one or two others had been present at that time, but it was eventually found that many others either heard or knew of the story.

They first suspect was opening bat, Jack Fingleton, a journalist by trade, who was present in the room and had to take the blame for it. Twelve years later, Fingleton, in his book, *Cricket Crisis*, seemed to be able to refute being that source. Bradman seemed the next most likely suspect. After all, he had a contract to write for the *Sun* newspaper and was friends with Claude Corbett. Corbett told others, including his daughter, he had met Bradman that night at North Terrace in Adelaide with the story. Bradman denied it.

We'll never know who the leak was.

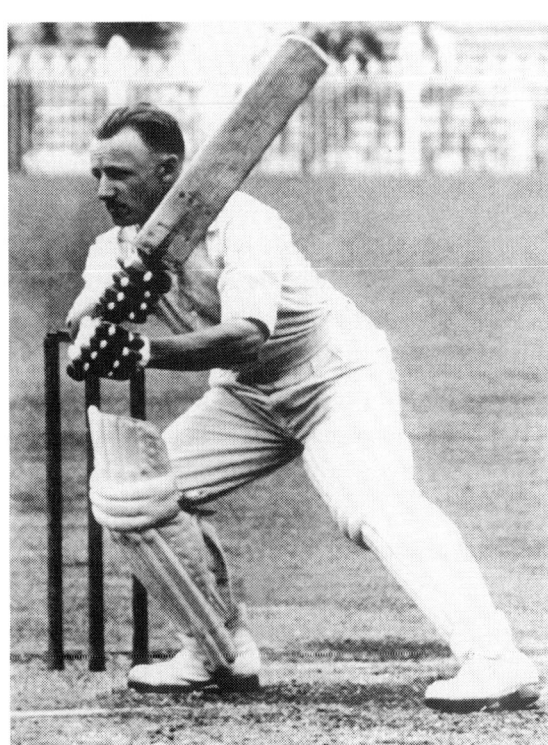

Sir Donald Bradman at work (AAP IMAGE/ S&G)

Pre-World War II was also a time, thankfully now a thing of the past, when there were Australia-wide divisions between Catholics and Masons. Bradman, a Protestant, Mason, Anglophile, Establishment man, could be contrasted with the Irish Catholic, rebellious, hard drinkers such as O'Reilly and his friends. There were tensions on the team. After the Third Test in 1936, with Australian two down in the Ashes series, four players were hauled up before the Australian Board of Control (now the Australian Cricket Board) presumably to question their loyalty and commitment to their new captain, Bradman. The four, however, did not include Fingleton, who was said to be the ringleader of the anti-Bradman faction. The meeting ended a complete farce when the Board was challenged by O'Reilly to put up or shut up. Those players always blamed Bradman for being carpeted. He denied it until the day he died and said he had not been informed that the meeting was to take place.

After the war, Bradman's younger team-mates, with one exception, idolised him, while he, in turn, described the 1948 tour as his happiest. His relationship with Keith Miller could at best be described as ambivalent, as will be discussed later. Many in that team were very disenchanted when a few years ago his 1948 team was feted at a dinner in Adelaide, and The Don did not attend. Bradman said he had a previous dinner engagement.

There used to be an argument, which always seemed a silly one to me, that he was not such a great batsman because he couldn't bat on sticky wickets in the days when pitches were left uncovered; yet another version was that he was not so great because he was not as graceful as other batsmen such as Victor Trumper. This theory was pushed enthusiastically by Jack Fingleton. I was with another ex-Australian Test captain, Jack Ryder, one day when the argument came up. Ryder was asked what he thought of the argument.

'No, no, he couldn't bat,' said Jack, sarcastically. 'He would just belt the shit out of any ball he could reach.'

End of argument!

It has also been claimed, with justification, that Bradman's tight-fisted uncompromising position with the players when he was on the Cricket Board had a great deal to do with their revolt in the 1970s, leading to the formation of Kerry Packer's breakaway World Series Cricket in 1977.

One controversy Bradman had to live with concerned his involvement with his one-time mentor and high-flying boss, Harry

Hodgetts, who had arranged his switch from New South Wales to South Australia in 1935. Hodgetts was, among other things, a member of the Board of Control, a member of the South Australian Stock Exchange and a leader of South Australian society. He not only paid Don a good wage and allowed him time off to play cricket, but also introduced him to his Stock Exchange business, where Don made rapid progress. Hodgetts gambled on the futures market, went bankrupt and was sent to jail for five years. Bradman moved quickly to take over the company, renaming it Don Bradman and Co. Rumours about how all that could have happened still circulate in Adelaide to this day.

It would be difficult to estimate how many books and articles have been written about The Don, or even how many more will be written, including presumably some warts-and–all versions about this complex character. There certainly seems no end to them.

BEING THE SON or daughter of a famous parent would have to be one of the most difficult things in life. Examples abound about such difficulties in famous families, especially in America with the likes of the Kennedys, Rockefellers and many movie stars. The problem is how the children are, or are not, managed as they struggle to find their own niche and establish their own personality. Most commonly, and for a variety of reasons, they are not handled at all well. Some children are over-indulged, some treated harshly, many are lonely and feel ignored, and many are misunderstood.

Growing up in a small, closed community, as Adelaide was in the 1950s and 1960s, must have presented John Bradman, the only son of Don and Jessie, with some real problems. He did play cricket for a while. He was also a fine athlete with a promising career as a hurdler, setting a State 120-yard hurdles record until a knee injury put an end to that. The first question people would always ask when meeting him was 'Are you Don Bradman's son?'.

John went to work at his father's stock exchange business, but was constantly being asked what his father would do in a similar circumstance, so he left. He also decided to leave home, but travel in Africa and England gave very little relief, as his name was still recognised. He went to Scandinavia where he knew no one would recognise him or his surname and was happy there for some time. In 1972 he changed his name to

Bradsen. Jessie told me and Monica that she could understand his wanting to change his name; Don said he could not understand it at all. He also suggested that if John was going to change his name, it might have been better to change it to something completely different. Another problem for Don at that time was that Sweden in those days was synonymous with so-called 'free love'.

Eventually, John returned to Adelaide as an Adelaide University lecturer in law, finding happiness with his other great loves, wine and jazz music. He married and had two children. It was a strange arrangement in that in the telephone book in those days, the two names Bradman and Bradsen were listed together.

There is a happy ending to this story. After a time, father and son reconciled and before Don died they had become very fond of each other, close friends. John says how very proud he is of Don and of his achievements. He also foresaw, and decried, the incredible degree of hero-worshipping and the iconic status that followed his father's death. He gave a beautiful eulogy at his father's memorial service. One particular phrase: 'He remained so astonishingly unimpressed with himself', could well have been his father's epitaph.

John changed his name back to Bradman.

'It's pretty hard to be serious about cricket when you've had a couple of Messerschmitts up your arse.'

7. NUGGET OF GOLD

KEITH 'NUGGET' MILLER was a true, genuine war hero with a name worthy of the title. When he was born at Sunshine in Victoria on 28 November 1919, his parents christened him Keith Ross after two famous Australian World War I pilots, Keith and Ross Smith. At the time the Smith siblings were leading in the London to Sydney Air Race, having set off from England 16 days before Miller was born. They were to go on to win the race, landing on Australian soil when he was just 13 days old. It was ironic that Keith Ross Miller would be a pilot in the next World War.

Miller was a natural sportsman. He played fullback for the Australian Rules team, St Kilda, before and just after World War II, but after suffering an ankle injury wisely decided to concentrate on his cricket, a sport he had shown immense promise in, helped by early tuition from his cricket (and maths) master at Melbourne High School, the former Test captain Bill Woodfull.

Nugget flew Mosquito night-fighters during the War and once crashed a plane saying, as he walked away, 'Nearly time to draw stumps that time, chaps.' Like all heroes, he was most reluctant to speak about any of his war exploits. Ask him something about it and he would place one finger to his lips. I think that this flamboyant, charismatic character, who was seemingly friends with everyone in the world, all on a first name basis, had quite a shy streak underneath it all. He could be a nervous wreck in the dressing-room before going out to bat and was quite a tentative starter.

That is also the reason why he failed so dismally when he hosted a television sports show when TV first started in Australia in 1956.

His charisma meant that he was one of the trailblazers for sportsmen endorsing products. How many young men bought Brylcreem because Miller said he used it on his massive shock of hair? Brylcreem … a little dab'll do ya! Brylcreem … you'll look so debonair. Brylcreem … the gals will pursue ya … when you're using Brylcreem on ya hair.

Miller would attract women as sure as flypaper attracted flies. I used to ask my wife, Monica, during the 1950s if she'd like to come to the cricket. The inevitable answer would be, 'Is Keith Miller playing? I'll come if he is.'

He was an imposing figure on the field whether batting or fielding. But it was his fast bowling that caught the eye. He loved to run his hand through his long, black hair as he walked back about nine steps. This may not have been because he featured in the ads for Brylcreem, but it certainly could have helped with getting more swing out of the ball. If he had just been hit for four he would clap impatiently for the ball, walk a few steps before suddenly wheeling around to let fly with a bumper.

Playing against England in the Victory Tests at the end of World War II, Miller came on to bowl against Denis Compton, the man who featured in the English Brylcreem ads. Compton had not seen him bowl

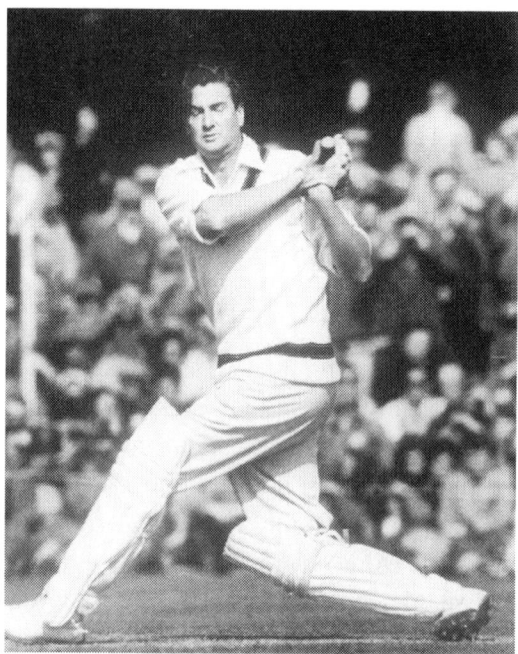

Keith Miller, a natural sportsman, and true hero
(AAP/SPORT THE LIBRARY)

before, so he asked the Aussie wicket-keeper, Stan Sismey, how his team-mate bowled. Stan replied he thought he was a bit quick. Miller came off a few paces and Compton did not even see the first ball. A bit quick! Compton said his hair stood on end.

Keith loved England, the English people and being in England, and I sometimes travelled with him during a Test series between cricketing venues. At the time he was writing for the *Daily Express* newspaper. Whenever possible, he would call into some cemetery where old Air Force mates were buried and pause to pay his respects and shed a tear. One special place for him was where he normally drank with friends in Bournemouth during the War. A German bomb had flattened it while he was away playing a match in London.

If the definition of an all-rounder is confined to those who could be chosen to play Tests for either their batting or bowling alone, then quite a few good all-rounders could be included in that definition. Each Test-playing country would have one standout nomination, chief among them would be Garfield Sobers (West Indies) and Ian Botham (England). Australia's nomination would surely be Miller for his batting, bowling and fielding.

Some very good observers, including CB Fry and Neville Cardus, compared his batting with that of Victor Trumper, especially after the 1945 'Test' at Lord's. Playing for the Dominions against England, in an innings punctuated with massive sixes, he scored 100 before lunch on the way to 185 in 165 minutes — it is an innings still talked about today. A lovely story is told about that innings. When Miller went out to bat he asked umpire Archie Fowler if it was true that only one player, Australian Albert Trott, had ever hit a ball over the Lord's pavilion. Fowler confirmed the fact, and Miller noted, 'Well, Archie, today I'm going to be the second.' Sadly Miller didn't manage to emulate Trott, but six times Miller belted the ball into the pavilion, and once the ball soared above the roof only to be stopped by a broadcasting box that wasn't there in Trott's time.

Subsequently, Miller's heavy bowling load, often having to bowl into the wind, eventually took the golden edge off his batting and he did not score as many runs as he might have done.

He had the most incredible memory of any person I have ever met. As he was the most popular cricketer of all time, everybody knew him and would come up to say 'G'day, Nugget'. He would immediately recognise each person and address them by name. I was once having a drink with him (that could well be a recurring theme) when a man walked up and said, 'You may not remember me, Mr Miller.' Nugget put his glass down and as his mind clicked into gear, replied, 'The West Indies, four years ago at the airport, and your name is …' Miller reeled off the guy's name (I can't remember what it was, for what that's worth). It was the first time they had met since then. This fellow seemed very impressed, not half as impressed as I was.

'Nugget, you must have set that up,' I said. But he hadn't. His memory also extented to a large record collection, and his great love, classical music. When flying over the Rhine during the War, he made a detour to look at Bonn because it was the birthplace of Beethoven.

Miller had a wry sense of humour and was known for his loyalty to his mates. One night we were attending a charity function with his great friend and bowling partner, Ray Lindwall. The compere was rabbiting on to the audience, 'Do you realise that we have with us two great fast bowlers who between them have taken 400 Test wickets?' Miller leaned over to Lindwall, and smiled, 'Congratulations. I didn't know that you had taken 30 Test wickets.'

Once, an ex-Australian cricketer, who had been working on the railways, was found with a load of railway equipment under his bed. The judge was not at all impressed with his explanation that he was keeping it there to mind for a friend. But Miller gave him a resounding character reference and quoted among other things Rudyard Kipling's poem *If*, saying that here was a man who had walked with kings yet never lost the common touch. When asked why he had done that when the accused had seemed so obviously guilty, Miller replied that he was a mate and he always had to stand by a mate.

He was captain of the NSW team, having moved to Sydney in 1947, and harboured visions of being Australian captain. But his idiosyncratic style didn't appeal to the heavies. He was appointed Australian captain for a game against Hampshire during the 1956 tour but arrived too late for the toss and Ray Lindwall had to stand in for him. He was the captain of the Manly cricket team when he came to live in Sydney after leaving Victoria. His appearances were fairly spasmodic, as he was away so much. Once he did play as captain for Manly, and a reasonably large crowd had turned up. He went out, won the toss, returned to the dressing-room, took off his cricket boots, put his feet up, turned the wireless on to the races announcing, 'You guys look after it. I'm too busy, so I'm not batting today.' The crowd was waiting expectantly for him to appear. Manly got to eight wickets down at the end of the day, but Miller still hadn't made an appearance.

He seemed to reserve his fastest bowling — and most of his bumpers, which could be quite lethal — for his best friends, such as Denis Compton, or a batsman he admired. He gave England's Len Hutton and West Indian Everton Weekes a terrible going-over. His attack in Sydney and Brisbane in 1951 against Weekes, with his partner in crime, Lindwall, definitely overstepped the mark. When chipped by the umpire, Miller replied with something along the lines of, 'You should have seen what we gave to Hutton.'

Miller's relationship with Bradman, both great crowd pullers, could, at the very best, be described as ambivalent. There was mutual respect and Miller recognised the genius in Bradman's batting and the contribution he made to administration. Although they both papered over any differences in public, they were highly critical of each other in private. They were very different characters. As might be expected, the flamboyant, dashing fighter pilot with the devil-may-care attitude to life, and the calculating, make-every-post-a-winner captain were differently motivated. Miller certainly

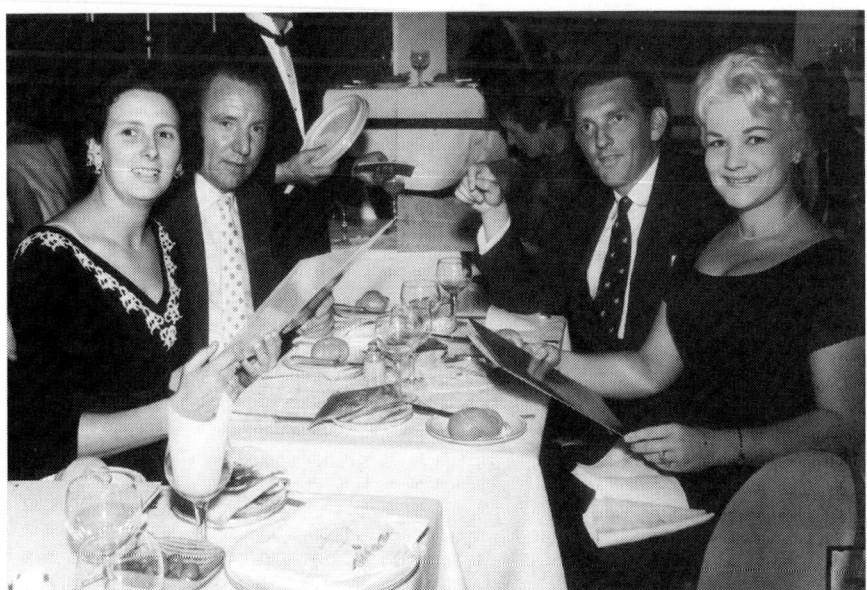

Having dinner with the Lindwalls, from left: Monica, Ray Lindwall, me and Peggy Lindwall, London, 1961 (BRIAN CORRIGAN'S COLLECTION)

resented being overbowled, especially on the 1948 tour of England. He had a back injury. It was not the usual one fast bowlers get, which is a stress fracture of a small bone in the lower spine. Miller's injury was the result of his airplane crash and was to trouble him on and off all his life.

Keith was critical of Bradman and his captaincy in two of his books written with RS Whitington, *Bumper* and *Cricket Caravan*. Not a very good career move if you wanted to remain in the Australian team and become its captain.

In later life, Keith suffered some serious disabilities. He had a slight stroke while at the Melbourne Cup in 1992 and fell, fracturing his hip. He was treated with a hip replacement and was told rehabilitation should be done through exercising. He took to the exercises enthusiastically, but there was a problem because the cup of the hip replacement was too large for his hip. He was in considerable pain, as might be imagined, but was told he was not trying hard enough and should exercise even more. He was in absolute agony until finally the problem was recognised and a proper fitting hip was inserted. This took a great deal out of him and he was ultimately confined to a wheelchair. Incredibly, in 2002, at the age of 83, he divorced his wife, Peg. They had been married since 1946.

A story that sums up Keith Miller and his relationship with Bradman: Bradman was ruthlessly determined to go through the 1948 tour of England undefeated, and had once told Miller he wanted him to grind England into the dust. It was an attitude that did not sit well with Miller's approach to the post-War game. Once, when Australia scored a record 721 runs in a day against Essex, Miller delivered his own judgment on such tactics by handing Trevor Bailey his wicket for a first ball duck. His captain was unimpressed.

But before that, after scoring a massive total in the first Test after the War, in Brisbane in 1946, Australia won by an innings and 332 runs. The ground was flooded after a violent storm, and England was twice caught on a sticky wicket. The ball jumped all over the place and the English batsmen took many knocks. Miller had cut his pace down and was lethal enough, but his captain kept asking for him to bowl faster.

The Don, not impressed, said to him later, 'Keith, you do not seem to take your cricket very seriously.'

To which Miller replied, 'Well, Don, it's pretty hard to be serious about cricket when you've had a couple of Messerschmitts up your arse.'

'The crowd seemed to melt away and here was I standing next to my hero. My tongue stuck to the roof of my mouth. I hadn't thought of a thing to say to him.'

8. NOT A CASE OF LUCK

WHEN I WAS at school at Joey's we had a mathematics teacher, 'Trigger', beloved by everyone, especially me. He was a real Mr Chips type. As well as tutoring us in maths he would also tell us stories about the War of the Roses. Not the real one fought out in the fifteenth century between supporters of the two Royal lines of York and Lancaster, but Yorkshire playing Lancashire at cricket.

Trigger was also the first to tell me the story about the little man who left his hat on the seat during a game to reserve his spot and when he came back he found a very large man sitting in the same seat. The little guy protested, but was told, 'It's bums not hats that keep seats around here.' It's a story famous Yorkshire fast bowler Freddie Trueman has since purloined as his own.

I used to think that if this great man (Trigger) could get all excited about a game being played over the other side of the world, there had to be a lot going for it. He sparked a love of cricket in me that became unstoppable.

One other thing I remember was him saying that Sid Barnes (I'd never heard of him then even though he had played one Test in England before World War II) would become the best batsman in Australia. I stored that snippet of information away and when Tests started again after the War, this opinionated teenager told his father that Barnes was a better batsman than Bradman. Although this confirmed my father's opinion that he was raising a simpleton — and nearly started another war in our household — I stuck to my guns. My mother had to intervene to prevent me from being thrown out of home.

Sid Barnes did turn out to be a pretty good opening bat and I was at the Sydney Cricket Ground in 1946 (I had pinched, borrowed is a better word, my father's member's card and wouldn't be alive to tell this story if he had found out) when Barnes scored 234, the same score as Bradman had already posted, but Barnes scored at a hell of a slower rate. Barnes then threw his hand away to stay on the same score as The Don.

After the 1948 tour of England, Barnes returned with a better Test average (some 82 to 72) than Bradman himself, and on his retirement was one of only a handful of Test batsmen who had averaged over 60. I felt justified in my claim, but soon found that this hero I had championed had feet of clay.

Barnes had a host of troubles with the cricketing authorities and in a way I am sure that suited him. At the stage I first met him face to face in late 1948 he was threatening to retire from cricket. One of the problems he had with the Establishment was he had brought back from England some home movies he had taken on tour and was now exhibiting them — for money. Shock! Horror! He put his show on at our local town hall and, as you might imagine, I was keen to go to see the grainy images. When the show was over there were some light refreshments and a large crowd milling around Sid. I realised I would never get close to him. As I was about to leave, a strange thing happened, the crowd seemed to melt away and here was I standing next to my hero. My tongue stuck to the roof of my mouth. I hadn't thought of a thing to say to him.

'Gee, Mr Barnes,' was the best I could get out. 'Is it true you are going to retire from cricket?'

'Listen, son, why don't you just read the newspapers,' he snarled as he turned away leaving me stranded. I went home and cried myself to sleep. This was the man that I had stood up for and who had nearly caused a family split.

Years later, Sid Barnes, his wife Alison and their two children, Sid and Helen, came to live near me and I used to see him as a patient. We became good friends and used to play squash together. Don't ask me who won because even though I reckon I was a better player, I was often cheated, no, let's not say it was cheating, call it gamesmanship. On one occasion I returned a drop shot and Sid sang out, 'You got that on the second bounce.'

'No,' I said, turning around indignantly, just as the ball bounced.

'Well, you just missed that one,' he said as he picked up the ball. 'My serve.'

And I didn't win the ensuing argument.

He used to ask me what car I was driving and I'd say a Volkswagen or whatever. He would then show me his late model huge American tank with a large speedboat in tow and tell me exactly how much it had cost.

Sid loved fitness training and jogging so I invited him to come down to Brookvale Oval when I was the doctor for the Manly Rugby League team in the mid 1960s. A couple of times, when Ron Clarke was in Sydney, I asked him to come down, too. Sid could not get over the difference in the fitness level between Clarkie and the Manly team and kept on telling them so in the newspaper column he used to write (or, at least someone else did, under his name).

One perfect day for me was when Sid asked the great Australian leg spinner Arthur Mailey and some of his old Balmain team-mates down to his place by the sea for the afternoon. It was a great afternoon with Arthur. He was a born raconteur, a genuinely funny man and a clever cartoonist. We whiled away the hours listening to his stories.

The immortal Victor Trumper had been Mailey's idol. He said that as a boy he had no money but would walk from Waterloo to the Sydney Cricket Ground just to see Trumper when he emerged from the Ground to go home. Could you imagine any kid doing that today?

As it turned out, Arthur's first game in first grade was against Trumper. In the first over, he conceded a couple of fours and then he had him stumped with a perfect wrong 'un that Trumper did not pick. What a great start to a career!

Mailey was a water meter cleaner when he was picked for his first Test in 1920. He finished his career with 99 wickets in 21 Tests, between 1920 and 1926. He titled his autobiography *10 for 66 and All That* after his career's best bowling figures, against Gloucestershire on the 1921 Ashes tour of England.

His last public appearance at the Sydney Cricket Ground was when he was granted a Testimonial Match with his friend the Test batsman,

Johnny Taylor, in January 1956. The pair, dressed in suits, walked to the middle of the field and the large crowd hollered for a ball to be bowled. Taylor shaped up with a bat and Arthur clean bowled him.

'I should have always bowled with my coat on', Arthur said.

Not long after the day at Sid's, Arthur died on New Year's Eve 1967, four days short of his 82nd birthday. Sid died six years later.

I treasure the memories of that wonderful day at Sid's seaside home when Mailey held us spellbound with his tales.

I WOULD THINK that all cricket lovers have a picture in their mind's eye about who was their favourite cricket player to watch. It would not necessarily be the best but one special to them. How could you pick one out of the dozens who could lay a claim to the title? Who among us wouldn't have liked to watch Trumper bat, if that had been possible?

My choice for a batsman would be Neil Harvey. All right, I can be accused of living in the past, but if so that is surely one of the beauties of cricket. With his twinkling footwork getting down the wicket, Harvey could murder an attack without looking like he would ever get out. When he retired in 1962, he had scored 21 centuries and 6149 runs, second only to the great Don Bradman (29 centuries and 6996 runs). Of course, quite a few other players have now surpassed these figures. Bradman played the least number of Tests to reach 1000 runs and Harvey is second on that list. Modern players have many more Test matches each year now in which to accumulate runs and centuries. And cricketers weren't looked after then as they are now and were usually left to their own devices to make a living.

There may have been a greater cover fieldsman than Harvey, but I doubt it. Later in his career he moved into the slips and again there may have been greater slip fielders than him, but I don't think he ever dropped a slips catch. Put the combination together and I am very sure there was never as fine a fieldsman in both positions. Without being mean, can you imagine that great slips man Mark Taylor patrolling the covers?

Harvey was surely the only man to walk when given out lbw when he was on 96, in a Test in Pakistan. There was one match in England in 1961 and rather unusually Neil was feeling distinctly seedy after a late night. The Australians were playing against Notts and Neil thought that the 50 he had scored contributed sufficiently to his team's effort. He was batting against a slow off-break bowler, Bryan 'Bomber' Wells when he hit the ball up in the air to cover and the fieldsman dropped the simplest of catches. Wells went off his brain and said, among other unprintable things, 'You always were the luckiest batsman in the world.' Wrong man to say that to.

'I'll show you how lucky,' said Neil. Ninety runs later he threw his wicket away for the second time … but this time not to Wells.

'Benaud ... looked and acted as if he had been anointed at birth to do this very job [captain Australia]. To the manor born, so to speak.'

9. RICHIE'S LAST BALL

I WANT YOU to imagine — and I must agree you will need an extraordinarily good imagination — that all the Australian cricket captains since World War II were together and able to vote on whom they considered to be the best of their number. (Oh, all right, I know that is impossible, but you know what I mean.) I have a sneaky suspicion that the winner of the poll would be Richie Benaud.

Should you try to dissect Benaud's attributes as captain, they may not differ to any marked degree from those possessed by any of the others. But he did seem to have them in a greater abundance, and he was a master tactician whose team would run through brick walls for him. This was possibly because he spent more time with them (today this is called 'bonding'), even with those who were considered not very successful. He knew them all and what they could do. The word 'attack' was emblazoned on his masthead in Tests or Shield games, so he proved to be very good for the game of cricket, which had been going through a particularly unexciting period at that time.

In 1962 we were living in England and all the talk in cricket was never 'How can we beat Australia?' It was always 'How can we beat Benaud?' I thought that was great, for they had developed a real Benaud complex. Many English critics claimed he was just lucky. Whenever I heard that excuse I always thought of the adage, 'Yes I am lucky, and the harder I work the luckier I get.'

Benaud attained the Australian captaincy through an extraordinary set of circumstances. He'd had some hopes of being made captain after Ian Johnson and Keith Miller retired in 1956, but the selectors gazumped him. The much younger Ian Craig, a man with great potential and public relation skills, was chosen instead. On the next tour to South Africa in 1957, his greatest mate, Neil Harvey, was vice-captain and Peter Burge was made the third selector, placing Benaud behind in the captaincy pecking order. He must have been disappointed, but never showed it, instead offering Craig great support.

In the winter of 1958, Ian Craig contracted hepatitis and was unable to play in New South Wales' first game. Benaud captained the side. Craig did play in the next two games, but was so seriously ill he really should never have tried to do so and he scored successive ducks. Neil Harvey, who had moved to Sydney, was then made captain for the next major game, a combined Australian XI against the touring MCC team. However, Harvey was not given a particularly good attack and lost that game badly, when spinner Tony Lock bowled into the rough made by the boots of fast bowler Fred Trueman. Nevertheless, it was expected Harvey would be announced as captain for the First Test, to be played two weeks later.

Through the field came Benaud, who immediately looked and acted as if he had been anointed at birth to do this very job. To the manor born, so to speak. He was always completely prepared to punt on his team's ability. If behind when batting or bowling, he would still insist on attacking. The first ball in his first Test as captain, bowled to opening batsman Peter Richardson, lifted off a good length, and Benaud immediately reacted by altering his field. Doesn't sound much, does it? But it was a signal that he was in charge and was prepared to change his field. His confidence and aggressiveness permeated the team. As did his excitement when a wicket fell, the new era of running to congratulate the bowler was born. Admittedly, it was not to everybody's delight at that time, but they came to learn to live with it.

He had never lost a series when he retired as captain and his teams bowled more overs in a day than any other. Compare that with the deliberate cheating that goes on still today with the go-slow tactics designed to starve the opposition of balls to hit.

Benaud was able to get the most out of Alan Davidson (a debt Davo has publicly acknowledged) who often seemed to have something

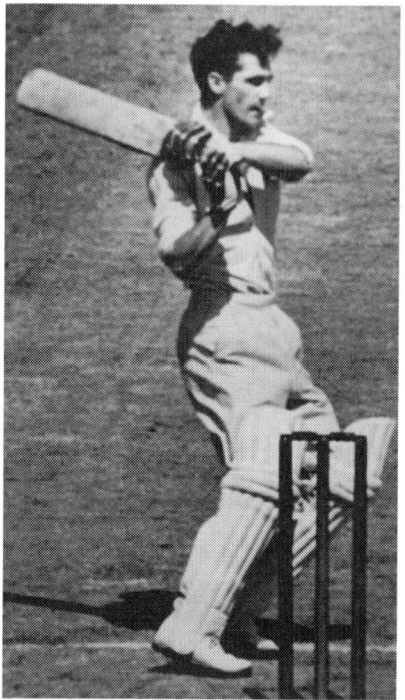 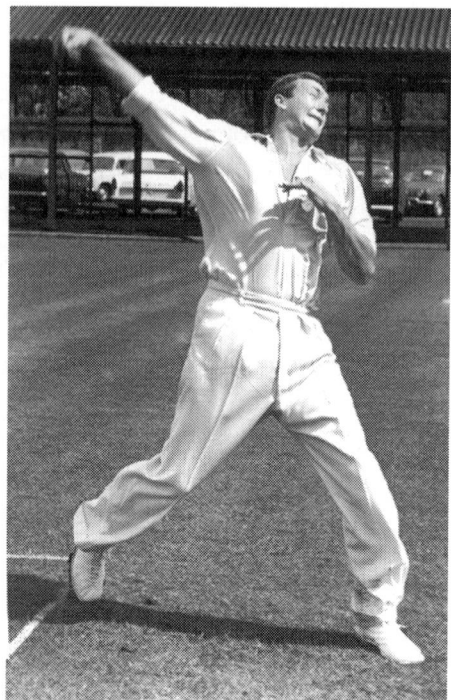

Neil Harvey (LEFT) was captain of an Australian eleven before his great friend, Richie Benaud (RIGHT). (BOTH AAP/ SPORT THE LIBRARY)

wrong that might prevent him from bowling. Davo, one of the greatest all-round cricketers ever to walk onto the field for Australia, once had a painful, swollen ankle injury.

'Al pal, I wouldn't try to bowl on that,' I told him.

'Don't tell Benords,' was Davo's answer. And bowl he did.

I love the story about Cammie Smith, who came to Australia with the great 1960–61 West Indies team as an opening bat, and was a real dasher. In the game against NSW, Cammie belted Davo all over the park and got to 48 in something like three overs. One ball he hit from Davo hit the fence so hard that it bounced halfway back to the wicket. Benaud had told his opening bowlers to give Smith some runs to try to con the West Indies' selectors into choosing him in the Test team.

'OK, Davo, that's enough, you can start trying now,' Benaud noted.

'What the bloody hell are you talking about? I've been flat out ever since the first ball.'

I SAW A fair bit of Richie in England in 1961 because on the first freezing day of the first game of the tour, he bowled a wrong 'un to Tom Graveney, and severely tore a muscle in his right shoulder. It was a very unusual injury. Benaud was treated in our department at UCH with Professor Alan Bass, using a series of newly devised shoulder exercises and stretchings. I would also sometimes do the treatments in his room at the beginning of the day. He couldn't bowl anywhere near his best until the Fourth Test at Old Trafford in Manchester, when he masterminded an Australian win.

That was his greatest psychological victory over England. His team was behind after the first innings by 177 runs, with all seemingly lost. Australia recovered in the second innings (including a last wicket partnership of 98 by Davo and fellow quick Graham McKenzie) to leave the English a target of just 256 runs. On the last day the swashbuckling Ted Dexter was thrashing us. But Benaud insisted they keep attacking, and on 76 Dexter snicked one and departed. England collapsed with Benaud taking 5–12 in 25 balls and finishing with six wickets. Australia won by 54 runs.

He was a great exponent of mind games. On that final day of the Test, England's last hope had rested with Brian Close who had a few swishes at the sweep shot, hit one six down the ground and was impatient to keep going. Next over, Normie O'Neill was told to swap his fielding position with a handicapped Ken 'Slasher' Mackay, and stand exactly ten yards behind the square-leg umpire. Norm may have been just a little confused, but Close most definitely was, for he hit the next ball in the air, straight to O'Neill who caught it. Benaud 1, Close 0.

RICHIE BENAUD WAS heavily involved in the formation of World Series Cricket (WSC) and asked me to become Australia's team doctor. In the 1970s the Australian cricket teams led by Greg and Ian Chappell had been seething with revolt at the way they were being treated by the Australian Cricket Board (ACB). The ACB was making a large amount of money with precious little of it filtering down to the players. The player's chance for change came with WSC, which started as a bitter dispute between Kerry Packer's Nine Television Network and the Australian Broadcasting Commission (ABC) over the rights to televise cricket. Players from all the Test cricket playing countries at that time were signed up with WSC.

Obviously details about its planning had to be kept clandestine. The wonder was that such a huge undertaking was kept a close secret for so long. Richie was approached early on by the Packer organisation to become their consultant and readily agreed. He was to introduce many innovations in both the rules of one-day cricket and television coverage, many of which are taken for granted today. One big advantage was that a decision concerning an idea or innovation would be made and acted upon as quickly as you could say 'Certainly, Mr Packer'. Things would take much longer to decide, if ever, by cumbersome cricket boards; a good suggestion might never get anywhere, sometimes because of the jealousy of other members. When authorities barred WSC from using the Melbourne and Sydney Cricket Grounds, wickets were prepared in trays under ideal conditions in Melbourne and then transported, often by helicopter, many kilometres to such places as the Sydney Showground, where a wicket had previously been non-existent. The first day/night game was played in Melbourne under lights using a white ball. But nobody who was there could ever forget the excitement of the next day/night game, played in Sydney, with queues so long that Kerry Packer ordered the gates to be opened to pack the large crowd in.

The South African-born, England team captain, Tony Greig, was also heavily involved in covert planning for the WSC, thus prompting the immortal words of John Woodcock, cricket writer for the English Establishment newspaper, *The Times*: 'Yes, but he's not English through and through, is he?'

Long-time friendships were dissolved in that bitter and costly dispute, and there were court cases between the cricket authorities and WSC. It always seemed there had to be an eventual compromise, and after two years they did get into bed together. And lived happily ever after? In the top ranks, yes, but in the lower ones, the deep scars took a long, long time to heal.

Richie's wrap-up of those WSC years, 'fun and frenzy', was typically apt.

BENAUD'S LAST TEST was against South Africa at the Sydney Cricket Ground in February 1964. The Test was drawn and Bob Simpson, who had taken over the captaincy, gave him the last over to bowl. When the team came off, the umpires had the ball and, as was their wont, tossed it into the box in the Australian room. I was watching and thought that ball would be a nice memento to keep, so went over and picked it up. Just then, Neil 'Hawkeye' Hawke — who ultimately played 27 Test matches for Australia as a medium pace bowler, and who had a most effective slower ball, a 'knuckle ball' derived from his baseball days — came up and asked what I was doing. So I told him.

'Oh, I really wish I'd thought of that … what a brilliant idea,' he said.

Well, I hadn't thought it was that brilliant, but when he asked how much I wanted for it, replied, 'Bad luck, Hawkeye, it's priceless.'

He went off muttering about the cruel injustices of the world. At breakfast next morning, there on the front page of the paper was a picture of Neil Hawke, with two beautiful blondes draped all around his shoulders, triumphantly holding up his prize — the last ball Richie Benaud ever bowled in a Test. But I still had that ball in my hand, and still have it.

I thought I would ask him next time I was in Adelaide where he said he had discovered the ball. But before I could get there he went to live and play in England for 11 years and did not return home until early 1980.

In July 1980 he developed an intestinal blockage, presumably due to scar tissue. The operation to fix it went horribly wrong. He developed peritonitis followed by an incredible number of complications. He was in a coma for three months, needed to be resuscitated 12 times after his heart stopped, and the operation scar burst open. He stayed in hospital for ages after all of that.

He had dreadful nightmares and hallucinations and told me he used to see an angel sitting on the bed. He attributed his unexpected survival to his wife-to-be, Beverley Myers, who nursed him with unbelievable skill and devotion day and night. The nice part of the story is that he and Beverley lived an enchanted life together afterwards. The sad part is that he recently died.

When I first saw him after his illness, I did not recognise him, he was so aged and scrawny, like a pale ghost. He told me that on many occasions, he knew he was about to die and had actually looked Death in the face. He talked about Fate and said that his favourite story was about the rich merchant in Baghdad who, while walking through the bazaar one morning, saw Death also walking through the bazaar. The merchant decided to flee and jumped on his horse to ride to Samarra, some miles away. Death turned to ask a bystander: 'Is that not the rich merchant?' Having been assured it was, Death said, 'That's strange, I have an appointment to meet with him tonight in Samarra.'

THERE IS ONE story about Hawkeye told to me by Neil Kerley, the Adelaide Australian Rules player who would appear near the top of everyone's list of the toughest men on a football field.

Growing up, Hawke was a sporting prodigy at both cricket and Australian Rules. In his first appearance in first-grade football, he had kicked about 18 goals. In his next game he had to mark Kerley. Hawke was greeted with a whack on his nose, breaking it. With tears in his eyes, he asked, 'What did you do that for? I'm only a kid.'

'Just to let you know you're playing a man's game now and I don't want you to forget it,' Kerley said he told the rookie Hawke. Kerley added dryly: 'His coach took him off a short time after that.'

The next time they met Neil Hawke was living in Perth. Playing for West Australia against South Australia, he was again marked by Neil Kerley. And the first thing that happened ... he was whacked across the nose.

Hawke said, 'What did you do that for? I didn't do anything.'

Kerley replied, 'It worried me that you might have forgotten the last one.'

THE CRY OF AN ITALIAN PROSTITUTE

At one stage, I travelled with the NSW cricket selectors to various country venues. In 1958 we went to Canberra, where a regional cricket final was being played. Canberra, then, could best be described as a small country town with its small population before its now vast army of bureaucrats was to become stationed there. Its cricket oval was quite picturesque but had few facilities, so we sat by the fence right at square leg. Soon after the second day of the match began, the Prime Minister, Robert Menzies (before he was knighted), whose genuine love for and deep knowledge of the game were well known, joined us. A short time after he sat down, one batsman played forward and was clean bowled.

'Middle stump,' I said, quite involuntarily.

'You could not possibly tell that from here, dear doctor,' the PM said.

I started to wonder if it had been correct when I saw the umpire pick up the fallen stump and hammering it back in between the remaining two stumps.

'Well, sir, I can assure you that I *can* tell from here.'

The batsman was coming through the gate and Mr Menzies called to him, 'Tell me, my man, how were you bowled?'

'Middle bloody stump,' he replied. No need for respect for anybody when you are bowled out, let alone middle stump, in front of the selectors.

Menzies did seem very impressed. The game finished early and he invited the selectors to go back with him to Parliament House for a drink.

'You must come, too, dear doctor,' he said to his newfound fellow authority on the game.

When we walked in the old white building, there was no evidence I can recall of any security, especially when you consider the degree of security you would be surrounded by and subjected to today. Menzies sat us down in his office and began to pour us beers. There were some family photos on his desk and two photos hanging on the wall, one was of a country scene, but the other was well known — a large autographed photo of Keith Miller; hair shining, athletic and imperious looking, as if carved in marble, making a glorious square drive against England at the SCG in 1950.

Menzies told the selectors about how he had once said to Test selector Jack Ryder that he should pick Slasher Mackay in his Test team. Ryder had replied, 'You pick your Cabinet, Bob, and I'll pick my Test team.' Menzies thought this a huge joke, saying something like, 'Try doing that in Russia.'

We were all getting on well and the PM spent the next two hours or so telling us stories, mostly highly libellous, about his political friends and foes. He would take off their voices, but especially those of Winston Churchill and former Australian Prime Minister Billy Hughes.

Menzies told one story about Hughes. At a dinner to mark his 50 years in Parliament one speaker alluded to the fact that Hughes often changed political sides for personal gain. He'd been in every political party except the Country Party.

'Yes,' piped up Billy, 'but you have to draw the line somewhere.'

Menzies also told a story about how the site for Canberra came to be chosen. It went on for quite some time, but the gist of it was this. At Federation in 1901, Federal Parliament was first housed in Melbourne, but the rules were that it had to be relocated approximately halfway between Melbourne and Sydney. An all-party committee was chosen to find the most appropriate location. Travelling was uncomfortable, good roads were mostly non-existent, it was a bitterly cold winter, it took far longer than they had imagined and there was no agreement among themselves about any of the sites, including the original spot, Dalgety, in the foothills of the Snowy Mountains. Relations were getting very frayed and there was talk of returning to Melbourne. So they were getting pretty desperate when they decided upon a large sheep station near Yass with the local Aboriginal name Canberra.

No sooner had they agreed upon their spot, than it had to be given a name. As each person in the committee had a favourite, the political infighting began all over again. There were some strange suggestions. One was to include part of the every state's name in the new name, another to call it Shakespeare. It came down to a choice of one out of two — Canberra or Myola. Most were inclined to favour the latter, but Billy Hughes, whom Menzies said he detested, championed the name Canberra.

In order to denigrate Hughes, the flamboyant American-born Tasmanian politician King O'Malley said, 'Canberra, Canberra sounds like a row of cans of beer.'

To which Billy Hughes replied, according to Menzies in his deadset imitation of Hughes's high-pitched, whining voice, 'Yes, yes, Canberra, Canberra does sound like a row of cans of beer. But Myola, Myola is the cry of an Italian prostitute.'

'After that, they all went home, and it was eventually called Canberra,' said Menzies deadpan.

SECOND OPINION

DOMINIC CORRIGAN

The son of Brian. After leaving school he joined IBM and eventually specialised in the financial side of leasing informational technology equipment.

SIMPLY THE BEST

GROWING UP AS the youngest (and only boy) of five children could well have created its own set of issues for me. It didn't. You see, having Brian Corrigan as my father gave me a free pass to every young boy's sports fantasy. It took me some time to realise that not every young kid has unlimited access to their sporting heroes.

My favourite memories, however, are not of meeting every single hero — though these are certainly right up there.

I clearly remember the 1968 Olympics, even though I was only four. I remember the photo of Dad holding Ron Clarke with tears in his eyes. Although I was too young to understand the full implications and nuances of the altitude story, I remember being very proud of my dad, getting his photo in the paper. Most of all, I remember the sombrero and toy car that he brought back from his travels to Mexico City. I remember him being away for a very long time, something I would certainly get more used to as I grew up.

About this time I developed a deep love for cricket, though I'm sure it was an example of conditioning and environment rather than of any innate ability or longing on my part. Dad was good mates with Test opening batsman Jim Burke, who used to come down to the nets with us and give me some pointers. In fact he gave me — and I still have them to this day — the batting gloves he wore in his maiden Test against England at Adelaide Oval in 1951, where he scored a century on debut (101 not out).

I remember 1972 and the Munich Olympics much more clearly, probably because I was four years older, and because of the terrible tragedy that befell the Israeli team at the time. I distinctly remember watching coverage of the closing ceremony, terrified that something would happen and that my dad may not come home. Shane Gould was the undoubted star of those Olympics from Australia's point of view, and I remember Dad presenting me with what he said was her poolside dressing gown, though I'm sure it wasn't.

It was also about this time that I really started to follow the Australian Test cricket side and actually understood the game. It was a very exciting time in Australian cricket. All of my early childhood heroes were from that '70's cricket side.

The year 1974 was certainly a stand-out. I was lucky enough to spend time with the great Socceroos, the only Australian side ever to qualify for the World Cup finals. I was basically their mascot, staying in the team hotel, going to training, chasing balls for them. It is hard to imagine in this day of total professionalism that you could get such access to the national side as a 10-year-old. I remember them all very fondly and can still just about recite their impressive win–loss record in making it to the finals. The biggest thrill however, was Ray Richards presenting me with his World Cup final shirt, Number 6, another treasured souvenir.

To alleviate the guilt associated with sending me off to boarding school for six years, Dad took me to Adelaide for the 1975 cricket Test against the West Indies. Even though I was young I remember the Adelaide Test being a great social occasion. I recall walking around the back of the Members Stand to find Dad talking to an older man. They were chatting and laughing, and obviously got on well. Every little boy would remember the moment that their Dad introduced them to Sir Donald Bradman. I was rendered absolutely speechless. I couldn't even muster a quick 'hello'. I did manage to shake his hand, again a fabulous memory. Normally, I would have got a clip on the ear for not speaking, but I'm sure that Dad understood that I was not being impolite. I was just awestruck!

Another wonderful memory for me was the whole World Series Cricket (WSC) saga. I was vaguely aware of the politics of the time, but all of my real heroes were part of WSC, and that was enough for me. Dad was the doctor for WSC in Sydney and as a 14-year-old boy I had access to the inner sanctum. I recall the first year where the Sydney Showground was used as the venue because the breakaway movement was not allowed in to the 'real' cricket ground next door. Mr Packer had set up a very nice private viewing area, and after a few days I had got to know the security guards so that I could pretty much come and go as I pleased. Cricket was a big part of my life. Imagine my joy when Martin Kent asked me if I would like to go to the nets and have a bowl at him and some of the others. I might as well have died and gone to heaven. Dennis Lillee took me aside and had a great chat about my bowling. I can only apologise to all involved for not having used all of this advice to better effect. Maybe it was a lack of talent on my part.

Having met all of these great people I can categorically state just which of them was, and still is, one of my greatest heros. Cricket legends Bradman, Lillee and the Chappell brothers come very close.

RICHIE'S LAST BALL

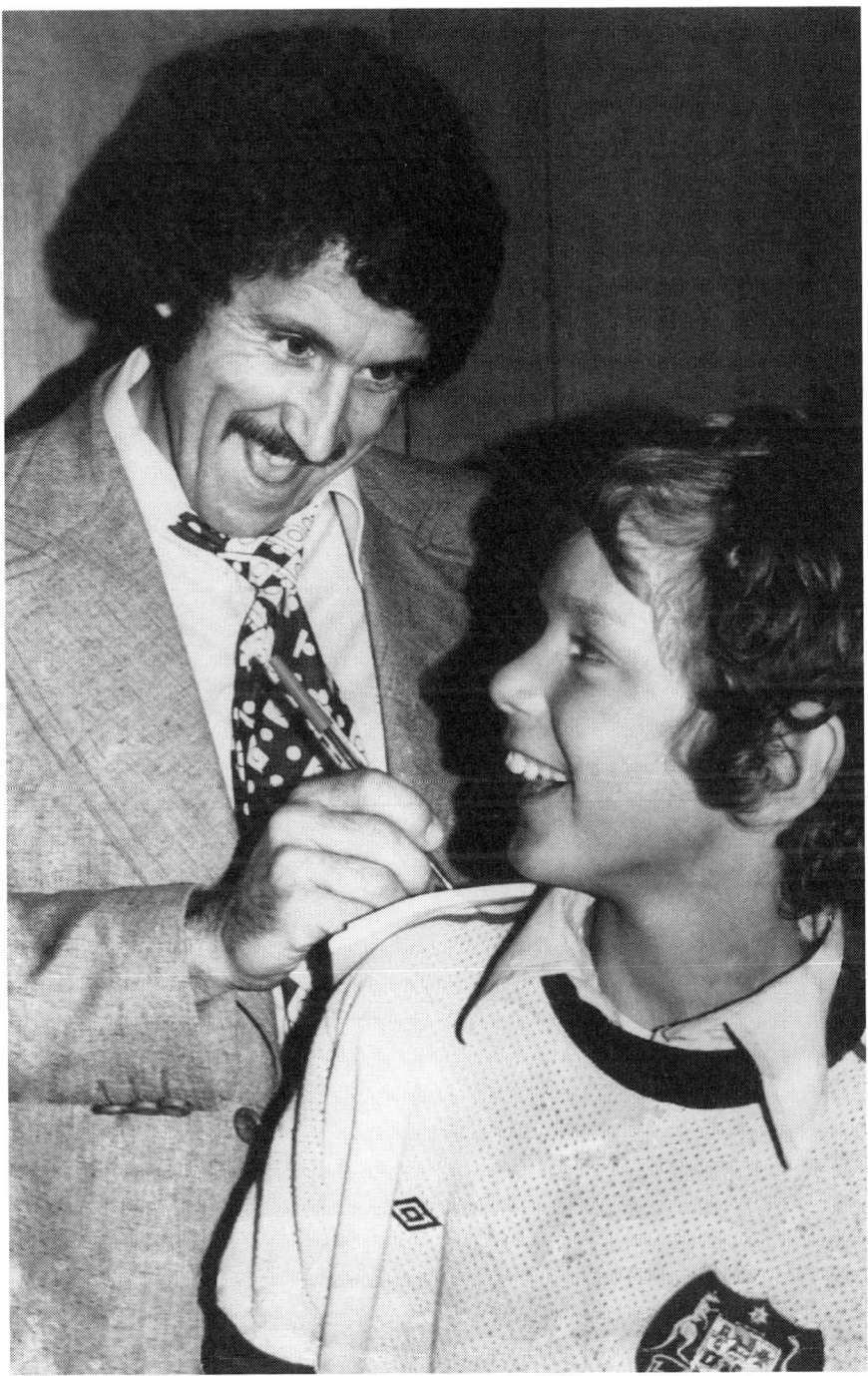

Soccer great Ray Richards autographing his 1974 World Cup shirt to give to my son Dominic (BRIAN CORRIGAN'S COLLECTION)

Socceroos Ray Richards and Johnny Warren are right up there. It was a great buzz to meet Viv Richards and Garfield Sobers, the West Indian cricketers. Soccer champ John Kosmina is remembered but for different reasons. And Jimmy Burke will always have a place in my heart. By quite a margin, my greatest hero is my dad. Despite all of the great sporting memories I have, when I quietly reflect on all of it, the greatest was the time when it was just me and him down at the nets at Curl Curl — he was Richie Benaud and I was Greg Chappell needing eight runs off the last over to win the Test match.

Brian Corrigan is quite simply the best Dad a boy could ever have!

'I became very confused with all his disjointed ramblings as he [Percy Cerutty] flitted from point to seemingly unconnected point.'

10. GENIUS OR RATBAG?

MUCH OF MY life in sports medicine has been devoted to assisting elite athletes. And moving among such stars one, quite naturally enough, comes into contact with their coaches — some quite brilliant and some legends only in the eyes of the media.

One of the most unusual was Percy Cerutty. It would be impossible for anyone to tell his life story without reference to the Olympic athletics champion Herb Elliott, just as it would be impossible to tell Herb's life story without including Percy. They existed in symbiosis, like bacon and eggs, peaches and cream, Ginger Rogers and Fred Astaire, Bogie and Bacall (or I suppose in modern jargon Posh and Becks).

Herb has described their working relationship as working together with two halves making more than one. He always said he could never have achieved his huge successes without Percy. Mostly this was due to Percy's ideas on life and training methods which struck a resounding chord in the young Herb's mind, allowing him to successfully undertake his huge training load.

I first met Percy Cerutty in 1960 when he was at the height of his powers just after Elliott's triumph in Rome when he had won the Olympic 1500m by about 20 metres from Frenchman Michel Jazy, in 3 minutes 35.6 seconds, an Olympic and world record time. Elliott's Olympic time was not to be bettered for 24 years. Soon after the 1960 Games, Herb, aged 22, retired undefeated in the 1500m and its metric equivalent, the mile, to study, be a family man and pursue careers in business and sport administration. Percy was shattered, but was unable to talk Herb out of his decision.

Percy had been born in 1895 into a Melbourne working class family and suffered chronic ill health. Despite this, he did become a passably good athlete for a time until 1939, when he suffered a severe depressive illness which devastated his life. Medical treatment in those days was decidedly unsuccessful as Percy soon found out and he decided to undertake his own rehabilitation from depression and phobias using a heavy exercise regime with weights, running, yoga and he became a health food nut. At about the age of 50, he ran an impressive sub-three hours marathon and also ran 100 miles in a day. He was an eclectic reader which helped him to develop his own credo, called *Stotan*, a mix of stoic and Spartan.

Percy has been called many things — an unorthodox innovator and motivator would probably be the mildest of them all. He was outspoken, eccentric, charismatic, touchy, idiosyncratic, egotistical, contradictory, and an exhibitionist who craved the limelight. There could be no middle ground with him — you either thought he was a genius or a raving ratbag. I came to believe the latter.

OUR PATHS DID not cross again until 1967. I had written an article for coaches about the problems associated with the altitude in Mexico City and Percy contacted me to say how much he enjoyed it. He said he believed altitude would be a huge problem for distance runners. Australians had nowhere to train at altitude but Percy, ever the enthusiast, suggested that Mount Kosciuszko, being our highest mountain and approximately the same height as Mexico City, might be the answer. So we arranged to take some athletes to the summit to run and I met him there.

The only thing that turned out to be in our favour was that it was summer time. My heart sank when I saw the conditions. There were no facilities and it was so rocky the athletes were more likely to do themselves some permanent damage than anything else. In the end it all came to nothing.

Percy did spend much of the time talking to me about his philosophy of Stotanism, with its emphasis on strength through communication with nature and the development of an inner force within us. He said that he had modelled his free-running style while watching Aborigines and animals run.

We also got talking about various training methods. Three possible training methods were available back then: interval training, circuit training and the Swedish Fartlek, or speed play. The latter was adapted by Percy to suit his rigorous lifestyle and the primitive conditions under which he lived.

It is difficult nowadays to realise how much emotion these different training methods would generate among anyone concerned with athletics. Their use was considered to be mutually exclusive; you had to be for one and against the others. It seemed to me at the time that this was a pointless argument, that the training method was relatively unimportant as long as it suited the athlete. The important thing was to be able to motivate the runner to succeed and no one training method could achieve that.

The method to be used was of importance to Percy, for his bitter rival, Franz Stampfl, was a proponent of interval training, which he (Stampfl) also claimed to have invented. Each coach loathed the other and the training methods the other used. For all that, Franz had many of Percy's characteristics. He was a larger-than-life character, tough, and wore a monocle. He also could be charismatic, individualistic, dogmatic, intolerant, a media junkie, confrontational, but dedicated and capable of motivating and inspiring his athletes. Stampfl pioneered the application of scientific methods of training in Australia.

Franz was born in Vienna in 1913. He hated Fascism and fled Austria to the United Kingdom after the Berlin Olympic Games in 1936. When war broke out in 1939 he was interned in England and, as an alien, he was shipped to Australia on the much-maligned ship *Dunera*. He was one of those now remembered fondly as the *Dunera* Boys. Stampfl returned to England after the War where he trained Roger Bannister to the first sub-four minute mile at Oxford in 1954. Soon after this success, he was invited back to Australia and set up camp in the Melbourne University campus. I used to visit him whenever I was in the Victorian capital in the late 1960s and 1970s and so got to know him fairly well. I was always most impressed with him and his training methods. He suffered a cruel fate when in 1980 while at the wheel of his stationary car, the vehicle was hit from behind and Stampfl broke his neck, leaving him to pursue a wheelchair existence. Yet he still continued to coach from his wheelchair until his death in 1995.

Getting back to Percy. It would be seemingly impossible to discover just how many athletes Percy actually did train or seriously influence for many deserted him after their initial contact. Percy claimed any athlete as his own if they had passed through his camp, no matter for how brief a time they were there. Even if they had left in disgust at his unusual

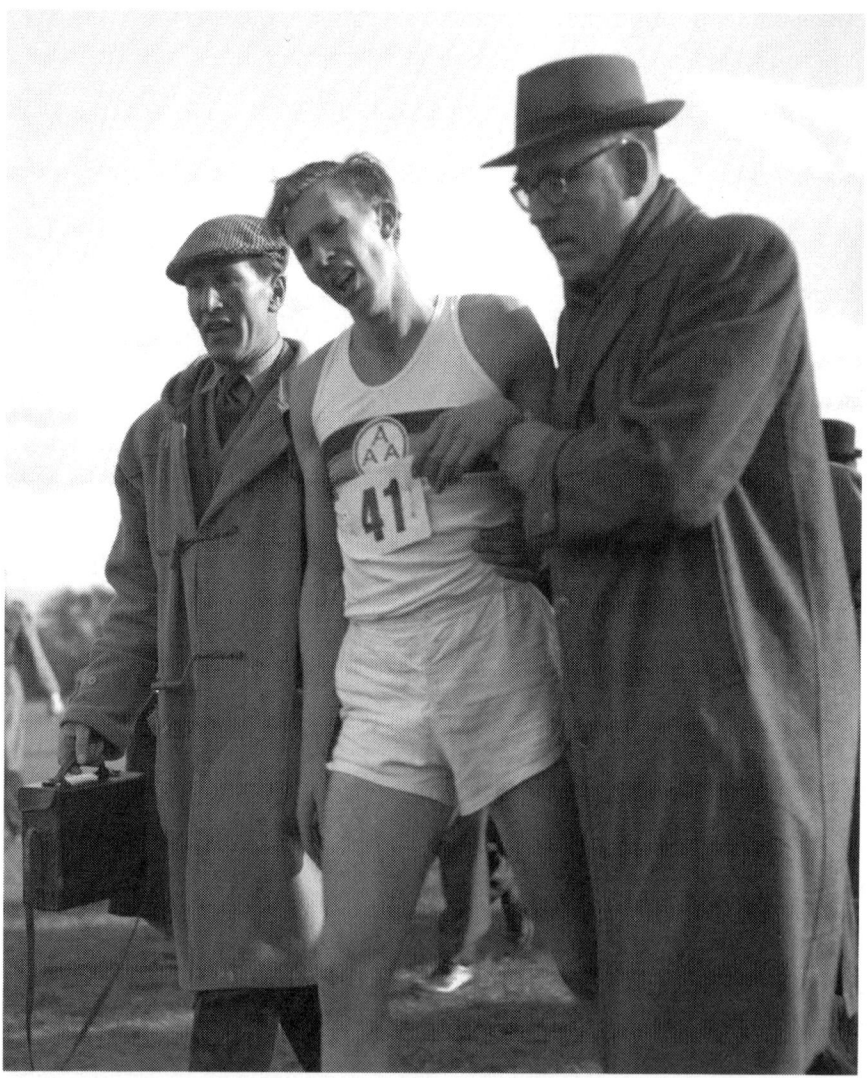

Franz Stampfl (LEFT) assists Roger Bannister from the track after he became the first man to break the 4-minute mile, Oxford, May 1954.

training methods or could not stand the pace, Percy still reckoned they were his. He told me that he had trained at least 30 world record breakers. He did train the great Australia runner John Landy from 1950 to 1952, but after a most disappointing time of 4 minutes 14 seconds in the 1500 metres at the 1952 Olympic Games, Landy decided to break from him and go his own way. After Landy became the second runner to break the four-minute barrier with a time of 3 minutes 58 seconds in 1954, Percy continued to describe him as one of his protégés.

One well-known athlete told me he had never met Percy until one day at the running track in 1969. Percy accosted him, waved his arms about wildly and shouted, 'Go on, go on, you can win this race.' When the athlete did so, Percy announced to all and sundry how the runner had won 'using my methods'.

Percy invited me to come and spend some time at Portsea, where he had built a shack to house his charges on the remote point of the Mornington Peninsula on the southern reaches of Port Phillip Bay, with its lovely surrounds of sea and sand. I looked forward to it with some relish. When finally I got down to Portsea, Percy was most courteous and seemed very pleased to see me. It turned out to be an unusual day. He had about 10 young athletes housed there and Percy, waving his arms around, told them to go off for a run and a swim. I thought that we would be spending a long time running around the sand dunes that were a feature of his camp, but we settled down to talk. Actually he did virtually all the talking, happy to have a captive audience to listen to his theories. Before very long, I became very confused as he flitted from point to seemingly unconnected point. In fact, I was never at all sure what the real point was. Consuming a bottle of sauterne may not have helped.

His sweet, long-suffering wife, Nancy, gave us lunch and towards the end of the day, I was invited to stay overnight. I had had more than enough and decided I would never make sense of any of his strange ramblings. He very kindly gave me two autographed copies of his books and I headed back to Melbourne, very disillusioned.

I never returned to Portsea.

'The villains in this story are the self-elected old men in the IOC itself. They chose to ignore all the warnings.'

11. BREATHLESS AND BEWILDERED

I HAD THE great honour and privilege of attending eight Olympic Games. Five times I was the Australian team doctor, once as medical officer for the Papua New Guinea team and twice through my involvement in trying to stamp out drugs in sport. My first Olympics were the most personally traumatic.

The Mexico City Olympics of 1968 were the first of the internationally controversial Games. Some of the problems weren't evident when the International Olympic Committee (IOC) awarded the games to the Mexican capital in 1963. The Olympic Games had never before been held in Latin America, and the IOC was keen to spread the gospel to that region.

There was always going to be difficulties because of the heat, smog and disorganisation due to *manana* (Spanish for 'tomorrow' and Mexican for 'any other time but now'). Beyond IOC control was a background of world problems:

- Because of apartheid in South Africa, some fifty nations threatened to boycott the Olympics if South Africa was allowed to take part. The IOC quickly capitulated and South African sportsmen and women were banned from competing. There were also arguments about the white regime in Rhodesia and whether it should be allowed to compete or not.

- Maoist student riots in Paris were leaving areas of destruction the like of which hadn't been seen since the end of World War II. On one day alone 10,000 students fought riot police in the streets of the Latin quarter, burning cars, overturning buses and leaving 600 injuries and more than 400 arrests.

- Prague Spring, the invasion of Czechoslovakia by the Soviet Union and its Warsaw Pact allies to stifle the democratic movement encouraged by Communist Party leader Alexander Dubcek. The defending all-round gymnastics champion, Vera Casavska, had been at the forefront of the fight for democracy as one of the high-profile signatories of the 'Manifesto of 2000 Words'. When the tanks rolled into Prague two months before the Olympics she went into hiding at a remote town in the Jeseniky Mountains and only emerged after the new Soviet-installed Government allowed her to go to the Olympics. She was an instant heroine, especially when she performed her floor exercised to the music of 'The Mexican Hat Dance'. She won four gold and two silver medals (to add to the three gold and two silver she ha won in Tokyo four years earlier). It was a real slap in the face for the invaders of her homeland.

- The corrupt Mexican government's brutal suppression of student unrest. As the Olympics approached secret police invaded a Polytechnic campus and many dissident students disappeared overnight. Student riots followed. Ten days before the Games were due to open there was a peaceful protest in the Plaza de las Tres Culturas. It mattered not to the Government that there was no physical unrest. Helicopters flew over the plaza and machine-gunned the unarmed protesters from the air. This was followed up by around 350 plain-clothes police snipers in buildings around the plaza. Between 250 and 300 students were killed and another 1000 injured. The IOC met in an emergency meeting to consider a suggestion the Games be aborted. In the end the Olympic chiefs refused to be drawn into the controversy, calling the slaughter 'an internal affair'.

For the athletes themselves there were two other major crises to be faced; both relating to their health.

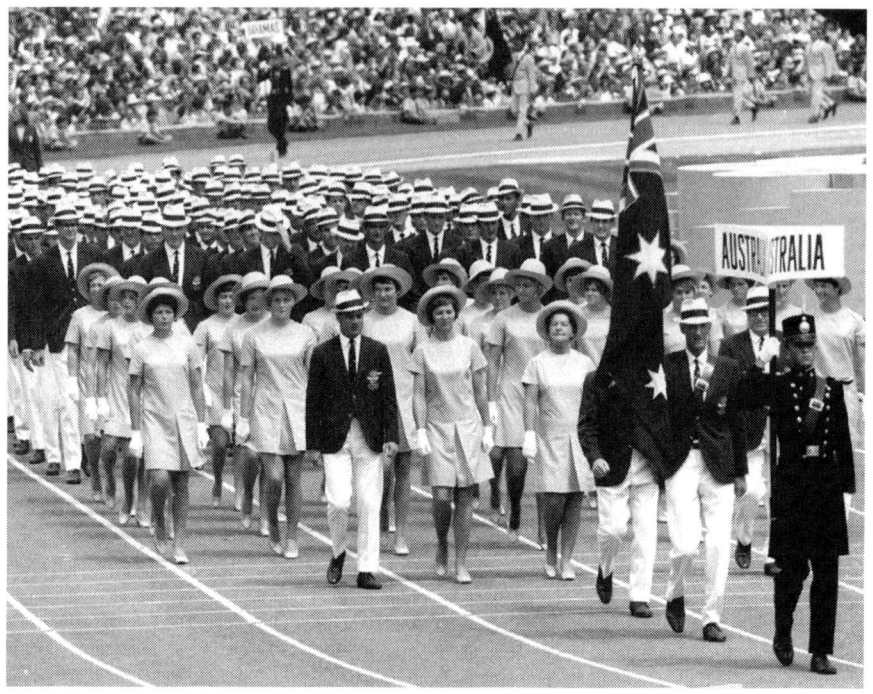

The Australian team at the opening of the Mexico Olympics in 1968
(AAP IMAGE/SPORT THE LIBRARY/PRESSE SPORTS)

First there was the problem of stomach upsets. The figures for stomach upsets among sportsmen and women competing in Mexico City were appalling. Two thirds of the athletes developed fever with either vomiting or diarrhoea, or both. One Australian radio commentator became very ill and, faced with the prospect of being treated in a Mexican hospital, he decided instead it was safer to fly home.

Infected water was the major cause of the illnesses. Those of us responsible for the health of the Australian competitors quickly decided peeled fruits and vegetables in salads were a strict no-no. There were also strong doubts about how often kitchen staff washed their hands, or if they washed them at all. Bottled water delivered to the Olympic Village in large flasks seemed to be the answer. We soon changed our opinion when we caught one of the delivery men filling bottles from a tap in the Olympic Village.

Members of the Australian team were given very strict instructions about how best to prevent, as much as possible, stomach infections.

They carried out our instructions so well that the infection rate was reduced to around 30 per cent. It was still not acceptable. But it was less than half the average of other teams.

The altitude of Mexico City was the greatest problem. Mexico City sat 2240 metres above sea level and this height reduced the air pressure. This meant that the so-called 'thin air' contained less oxygen. Since oxygen cannot be stored in the body, its only source is from the air inhaled. Normally, the oxygen content of the air at sea level is 21 per cent. At the altitude of Mexico City it was approximately 16 per cent. That's a reduction of almost a fifth. The body normally has some mechanisms that allow it gradually adjust to this reduction in air pressure, but this acclimatisation may take quite a while.

Some critics claimed we exaggerated the problems of altitude. The answer to their accusations is simple. Take a plane to Mexico City and check it out yourself. When you first arrive, there are no real problems when you take a leisurely walk around. Indeed, it may even feel invigorating, just as it does on our own Mount Kosciuszko. Try going for a fast jog and see how long it takes you to become breathless. Not long at all.

Some senior Australian Olympic officials were among those who were sceptical about our predictions. 'It's all in the mind,' they would say, echoing the misinformed Mexican Olympic chiefs.

They all started to change their minds when the horses for the equestrian events became so out of breath they refused to jump over their hurdles. We asked these doubters what the psychological hang-ups of the horses were. There was a classic case in the riding leg of the Modern Pentathlon when a horse called Ranchero had stubbornly baulked three times at one of the obstacles, ruining any chance of one of the favourites for a medal, West German Hans-Jurgen Todt. The West German was so angry he had to be restrained from physically attacking the horse.

The villains in this story are the self-elected old men in the IOC itself. They chose to ignore all the warnings of sports medicine specialists and respected scientists from around the world for purely political reasons. It's true that some of the warnings were overly dramatic. One Swedish professor claimed; 'There will be some who will die!' But such hyperbole was probably necessary to get the stubborn, misguided old Olympic chiefs to open their ears.

One fine English distance runner, Bruce Tulloh, a former European 5000 metre champion, retired before the Games started rather than risk his health. Protests from such respected people were simply ignored.

Why did this happen? The IOC preferred to listen to the Mexicans who deliberately ignored the mountain of evidence that predicted problems associated with altitude. 'No problem, Signor,' they would smile as they answered each and every query. The Mexicans even took foreign officials to Acapulco, the venue for the yachting, to show there was no problem. For heaven's sake! Acapulco is at sea level.

The IOC chiefs still stuck their heads in the sand after a British scientific team visited Mexico City in 1965 and proved conclusively there would be troubles ahead. Its tests on athletes showed a cut-off point of 2 minutes before the problems would be evident. In other words, all events of 1500 metres or more would take longer to run. On the other hand, the sprinters would benefit. Less atmospheric pressure and less air resistance would mean that sprint times would improve. So, too, in field events such as the long jump, records would be easier to beat.

To prove our theories, those of us involved in the medical well being of the Australian athletes sent a document to the Australian Olympic Council predicting the winning times in various events at the Mexico City Games. The Australian Olympic bosses were unmoved and toed the official line.

The same British scientific team also showed that it would take a minimum of four weeks for most of the athletes to acclimatise to the high altitude. In the case of those competing in longer events such as the marathon, the 20-kilometre and 40-kilometre road walks, and the cycling road race, it would take several weeks more. It wasn't a case of saying that if you run a marathon at this altitude you would die. It meant your time in that marathon would be about 2 minutes slower than normal and attempts to match sea level times might prove fatal.

The blinkered, narrow-minded IOC boss Avery Brundage compounded the error by announcing that, in order to preserve their amateur status, athletes *could* train at high altitude, but *not for more than four weeks* in any one year. This four weeks would include the time spent in Mexico City before the start of the Olympics. Australia complied, but most other countries turned a blind eye to Brundage's decree. The Soviets had a special camp high in the mountains near Alma-Ata (now

Almaty), the then capital of Kazakhstan. The Americans had one in the Rocky Mountains of Colorado. The French build an excellent sporting facility at the ski resort of Font Romeu, nestled around 2000 metres in the Pyrenees, near the Spanish border. The great Australian long-distance runner Ron Clarke went there to train for the Mexico City Games, but Brundage's decree meant he could only stay for less than a month. The French athletes stayed a lot longer.

The 1968 Olympics should never have been staged at such an altitude. So many athletes in distance events were unfairly penalised. Those who lived and trained in high, mountainous countries such as Kenya, Ethiopia and Mexico had a huge advantage because they were acclimatised. At Mexico City a Tunisian won the 5000 metre from two Kenyans (in a time almost a minute slower than Clarke's world record), it was gold to Kenya and silver to Ethiopia in the 10,000 metres (almost 2 minutes slower than Clarke's world best), an Ethiopian won the marathon and Kenyans finished one-two in the 3000-metre steeplechase.

In the end no athlete died but it was appalling to see so many elite sportsmen collapse. In one day no less than eighteen rowers were laid out. On another day half the competitors in the Modern Pentathlon collapsed.

And the worst affected of all those competing in the Mexico Olympics was Ron Clarke. The greatest shame of the Mexico Olympics is what happened to Clarke. It is testimony to the abject ignorance of the IOC.

'I burst into tears. I couldn't help it ... here in my arms was this great athlete who virtually had to kill himself in order to prove that these Olympics should never have been held.'

12. A BROKEN HEART

THE TRAGIC TALE of Ron Clarke at the Mexico City Olympics has been written many times before, but the full story has never been revealed until now.

Ron Clarke is arguably the greatest distance runner of all time. He set no less than seventeen world records during his career and at one stage, before the Mexico City Olympics, he held every world record from 2 miles to 10,000m. As a youth he had hoped to become an Australian Rules player with Essendon, joining his beloved brother Jack, the legendary footballer who played 263 games for the Bombers and starred in two grand final wins. A severe finger injury put paid to Ron's footballing dreams.

As a young athlete, Ron Clarke held junior world records for the mile (1609 metres) and 3 miles (4826 metres). He became part of Australian sporting folklore by lighting the Olympic flame at the Melbourne Cricket Ground to herald the beginning of the 1956 Olympics. As he circled the arena and climbed to the cauldron he was showered with sparks from the torch he was carrying and suffered painful burns. Soon after, he retired from athletics to concentrate on his career as an accountant and focus his very successful and enduring partnership with wife Helen and their three children.

Clarke sorely missed his running and made a comeback a year before the 1962 Commonwealth Games in Perth. He set the pace in the

3-mile event but was run down by New Zealand's fine distance runner and reigning Olympic 5000 metre champion Murray Halberg. And Clarke failed to finish the 6 mile race. In December the following year Clarke set the first of his world records in the 6 miles (9652 metres) and the 10,000 metres.

Clarke set himself a gruelling task at the 1964 Tokyo Olympics, competing in the 5000 metres, 10,000 metres and marathon. He led for much of the 5000 metres only to fade to ninth behind the surprise winner, American Bob Schul. As world record holder, in the 10,000 metres he tried to burn off the opposition by surging every second lap. The tactics seemed to work with all but four of his opponents out of contention by the halfway mark. In a rough and tumble finish, with lapped stragglers getting in the way, he was passed by the relatively unknown part-Sioux American marine Billy Mills and Tunisia's Mohamed Gammoudi and had to be content with the bronze medal. Then, in his fourth race in a week, Clarke tried in vain for a marathon gold. He led early but was pulled in by the defending champion, the great Ethiopian Abebe Bikila, at the 15-kilometre mark. Bikila went on to win, while Clarke slipped back to a credible ninth.

On a tour of Europe and the United States the following year Clarke set eleven world records in just sixteen appearances. Once again, this great form did not carry over into the 1966 Commonwealth Games in Kingston, Jamaica. He was beaten by Kenyans in both the track distance events; by Kip Keino in the 3 miles and Naftali Temu in the 6 miles.

There seems no doubt that Clarke's greatest disappointment in athletics was missing out on an Olympic gold medal. Theories abound as to why he didn't manage that elusive honour. Some critics claimed he could run only against the clock and not against other runners. In many races some opponents, such as the Kenyans, would run as a team, dictating tactics such as just when and who would take on Clarke at the front. Other detractors reckoned he was too nice a guy, or that he lacked guts. They said he lacked the killer instinct that champions like Herb Elliott would show in their races.

I remember a famous race in Melbourne in 1956 when Clarke slipped and fell. Our first sub-four-minute-miler John Landy, one of nature's gentlemen, was forced to hurdle Clarke as he lay on the track. Landy stopped, went back to make sure Clarke was all right, helped him to his feet and then, despite letting the entire field get what should have been a winning break, set off and won the race. Marvelling, I turned to one noted athletics authority and said, 'What a wonderful gesture of sportsmanship.'

'Sheer rubbish!' came the curt reply. 'That sends the wrong message. Only the tough survive out there. Landy should have run right over the top of him, spikes and all, to teach him how tough it really is.'

I believe all the various theories were wide of the mark.

Ron Clarke was probably the last of the true blue amateurs, one who loved his sport and ran for the sheer passion of it and the satisfaction it gave him. His motivation was running, not money. That is not to say he didn't make any money out of athletics. For all I know he may have made a considerable amount. He would run against anyone in the world, at any time and over any distance, even if it was not his favourite. Indeed, organisers of athletics meets would often change the distance to suit the local champion. It happened once in France when the distance was suddenly changed from 5000 metres to 2000 metres to suit the Frenchman Michel Jazy, the 1960 Olympic 1500 metres silver medal winner. It didn't matter to Clarke. The Australian ran and beat Jazy.

I believe Clarke had wanted Olympic success but on his own terms, without the help of a coach. He did consult two coaches early in his career — the eccentric Percy Cerutty and the down-to-earth Austrian Franz Stampfl (see *Chapter 10 — Genius or Ratbag?*). Predictably, Clarke's association with the eccentric Cerutty lasted one day.

The Austrian-born Stampfl was already a world renowned coach when he came to Australia in the mid-1950s. He had coached at Oxford where three of his star pupils, Roger Bannister, Chris Chataway and Chris Brasher had been involved in the race on 6 May 1954 that saw Bannister run the first sub-four-minute mile. Clarke and Stampfl split after only a year or so early in his career, apparently over training methods.

I am sure Clarke needed someone other than himself, who could help him peak for a particular race and plan suitable tactics for that race. The big problem, when he missed gold in the 10,000 metres at Tokyo in 1964, was that he didn't peak for the race and treated it just like an ordinary event at some obscure track and field meet. Clarke didn't analyse the opposition either. He later admitted that although he had met and admired Mills, a half Sioux Indian who had been raised and educated on a reservation, he did not consider him a threat in this race.

CLARKE *DID* FORMULATE a definite plan for the 1968 Mexico City Olympics, and like all good plans the main attribute was simplicity. Clarke had consulted Stampfl who pointed out the obvious, that Ron was the world record-holder for 2000 metres, 5000 metres and 10,000 metres and running as well as he had ever done in his whole career. The first event in Mexico City would be the 10,000 metres, Clarke's favourite distance. Stampfl told Clarke to run the first 8000 metres at an even pace, not worrying about the other athletes, then to go as fast as he could over the final 2000 metres — remembering all the time that he had run this faster than any man in history.

Ron loved the plan and tried it out successfully in a race in Sydney. He was also acutely aware of the problems of altitude and the lack of oxygen. He had gained some personal knowledge when he visited the Mexican capital in 1966 with his good mate and confidant Dr Zim Zimmerman, the Melbourne GP who was also the Essendon football club's doctor.

It was quite intriguing that Clarke was regarded by the athletics world as favourite for gold even though he was to be confronted by the problems of altitude and competition from the so-called 'Mountain Men'. Realistically, he would need a miracle to win at what was expected to be his last chance at Olympic success. And so it turned out. There would be no miracle. And the trauma of Mexico City would end his illustrious career.

The 10,000 metre event was held on the first day of the track and field competition, and it was soon obvious that all the warnings that the IOC had chose to ignore were proving spot on. A third of the runners collapsed, including the great Kenyan Keino (although to be fair, it was not so much because of the altitude but from stomach cramps).

If it hadn't been so serious it would have been comical. There were all these Mexican stretcher-bearers suddenly running all over the arena picking up the prone bodies of collapsed athletes. At one stage a quite rotund stretcher-bearer suddenly fell in a heap and had to be carried off himself.

Throughout this chaos Clarke was sticking to his plan. The lead had changed constantly and with 800 metres left there were only four runners left in contention — Clarke, running strongly, Mamo Wolde (Ethiopia), Temu (Kenya); and Gammoudi, the Tunisian who had won silver in front of Clarke at Tokyo.

With one and a half laps remaining those of us sitting up in the stands noticed a sudden and dramatic change in Clarke. He became as pale as Banquo's ghost, had visibly slowed and appeared to be unable to run straight. (Later it was revealed he was having trouble focusing.) His sight was blurred. He had, of course, run out of oxygen and was semi-conscious. How he ever managed to finish the race remains a mystery. But finish he did! Temu, the 23-year-old Kisii tribesman, raced past him, beat off Gammoudi and then Wolde to take the gold medal — the first Kenyan to ever achieve that honour. Significantly Temu's time was around two minutes slower than his best at sea level.

It took an incredible effort of will on the part of Clarke to complete the race in sixth place, the first non-altitude runner to finish. His willpower was greater than I could ever imagine. 'I had to finish,' Ron told me later. 'It was a question of pride.' He collapsed quite dramatically right under the IOC sign at the finish.

My immediate instinct was to get onto the arena and to Clarke's prone figure to see if I could help him. It was easier said than done. Running onto the field was not only prohibited but the arena was protected by a deep moat. How I managed to cross that moat I honestly cannot remember. I knew I had to get to Ron's side.

When I reached him he was completely unconscious — and remained like this for at least an hour. After giving him oxygen and making sure he was comfortable, I wondered what I should do next. Hospital seemed the obvious place, but the thought of a Mexican hospital definitely did not appeal, especially as Jim Howlin, the co-manager of our athletics team, had already died from a stroke in the hospital designated for our use.

As I knelt there wondering about the futility of the whole situation and contemplating my next move, I burst into tears. I couldn't help it as I realised that courage alone would never be sufficient to overcome the problems caused by the stupidity of the IOC. Here in my arms was this great athlete who virtually had to kill himself in order to prove that these Olympics should never have been held here. The heart of a trained athlete is the strongest muscle in the body, but nobody had considered what running with a lack of sufficient oxygen could do to it. I wasn't Robinson Crusoe that evening; many watching the drama from the stands told me later that they had cried too.

A BROKEN HEART | 91

AFTER A WHILE, my good friend Ray Weinberg, the Australian team's athletics coach, appeared. He had been held up going the long way through a tunnel under the moat. After Ron began to stir, we managed to get him to his feet and stagger our way to the medical centre. As he lay on a couch, Ron uttered his first three words, the classic 'Where am I?' Ray and I were relieved he had snapped out of his coma. Just then a tiny, mild-mannered individual arrived on the scene. He was very apologetic as he explained he had to perform a urine test on Clarke to test for drugs.

Now, Australian sports medicine officials had been at the forefront of those pushing for and organising drug testing at the Olympics. Only the year before had the IOC finally seen the light and begun outlawing performance-enhancing drugs. The Mexico City Games were the first where tests were taken. How anyone expected to obtain a urine test from a semi-conscious runner was beyond my comprehension. As it turned out, Clarke was unable to pass urine for several hours.

In this emotion-laden atmosphere I exploded. I loudly questioned the mild-mannered man's parenthood and sanity, but it all went over

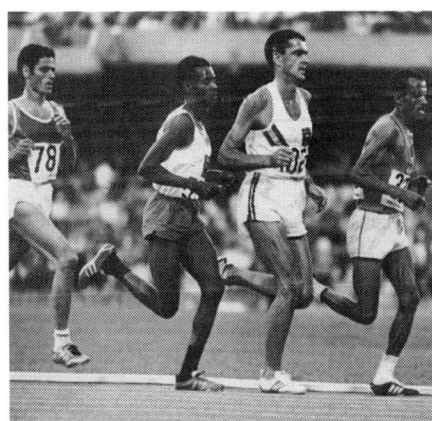
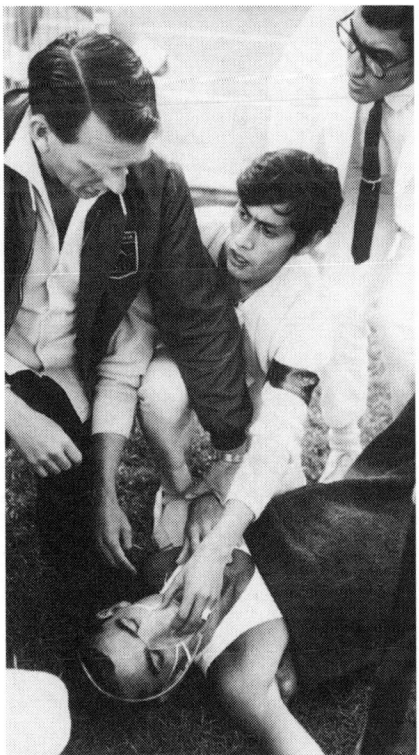

Ron Clarke running the 10,000 metres at the Mexico Olympics (ABOVE) and immediately following his dramatic collapse (BRIAN CORRIGAN'S COLLECTION)

his head. He was determined and said he would not leave Clarke's side until he had his test.

The one good thing this official did do was to organise an ambulance to transport Clarke back to the village. By this time we had been joined by Melbourne journalist Alan Trengove, a good friend of both Ron and me. We four Aussies squeezed into the ambulance for the trip, together with the little man and his urine testing equipment. It transpired that he was Professor Arnold Beckett, the head of IOC drug testing. We were to meet many times in the ensuing years and he would always greet me with the words, 'What about that time you tried to throw me out?' (I should point out that the persistent Professor Beckett did eventually get his urine sample, but it was in the early hours of the morning after the race. He had to follow Ron around for many hours before that important tinkle.)

The scene outside the Australian headquarters when we arrived back in the village was absolute bedlam. There seemed to be hundreds of reporters and photographers from all around the world demanding to talk to Clarke or to get his photo. They were jostling each other trying to get an advantage. The one question they all wanted answered was the one that had been preying on my mind during the journey from the stadium. Would Clarke be running in his heat of the 5000 metres in two days' time, and in the final two days later?

I told them that I honestly couldn't give an answer until we assessed Ron's condition the next day. This appeared to satisfy the throng, and that's the story every reporter wrote — except one. This fellow, who I had always regarded as a friend, wrote that Clarke was going to run against his doctor's orders, and he could very well die. I have never spoken to that journalist again.

By this time, Ron's wife, Helen, had telephoned from Australia in tears asking what we were going to do for him. I poured myself a very stiff whisky. It didn't really help. I tossed and turned in bed all night worrying about what was going to happen to this courageous Aussie athlete.

THE NEXT MORNING I was organising a cardiograph for Ron when the door burst open and in came a Russian sports medicine professor by the name of Seminov. He was a giant of a man with hands bigger than hams.

He wrapped one monstrous arm around my shoulders and announced dramatically, 'Ron Clarke will never run again!'

'Why?' I asked.

'Because he is deficient in Vitamin C,' came the reply.

Oh, really! Of all the problems that Ron could or did have, I was quite certain that a Vitamin C deficiency was not one of them. But now was not the time to argue. I thanked the big Russian. He smiled as he unwrapped his massive arm from around my shoulders and left.

Ron decided when next he would run. He told me that morning that, although he felt a bit weak and tired, he would be able to run the heat of the 5000 metres the following night. I had serious doubts. There was no way he could have a trial run to see if he was OK, but I had a plan. The first five finishers in the heat would qualify for the final and there was really only one good runner in Ron's heat, Temu, who had won the 10,000 metres. I suggested Ron take it easy and finish fourth or fifth. That way we could use the heat as a test to see whether he could stand up to a torrid 5000-metre final.

'Good idea,' said Ron. 'Let's do it.'

Under the archaic rules in Mexico City, it was forbidden to take an athlete from the village to the stadium by car. I managed to convince the Mexican authorities that I needed a car and was able to take Ron with me. As we drove to the stadium the tension in the car was obvious. The cliché — you could have cut the atmosphere with a knife — was the only way to describe the ambience. Neither of us spoke a word. I kept wondering whether I had been right in letting Ron try for the 5000 metres after such an ordeal two days earlier. I speculated as to what Helen would be thinking. As we drove through the gates into the stadium, Ron suddenly blurted out, 'I can't do it. I just can't do it.'

'You can't do what?' My first thought was that he had decided not to run at all.

'I can't run in any race and not try to win it. I have to run to win. I can't run to finish fifth.'

So much for my plan! Considering all the circumstances, it was easily the most courageous decision I have ever known in all my years in sport. Ron ran that race as he had promised and was just ahead of Temu as the finish line loomed. Ron paused for a moment as a mark of respect to Temu and they crossed the line together. Clarke lined up the following day for the final, even though he was obviously quite unwell. History shows how he finished fifth, just 7.4 seconds behind the winner, Tunisia's Gammoudi. Once again Clarke was the first athlete who wasn't from a high altitude environment to cross the line. Trailing Gammoudi were Kenya's Keino and Temu with Mexican Juan Martinez fourth. The winning time was 48.4 seconds, slower than Clarke's world record.

It was the last time Ron Clarke competed at the Olympics. His dream of gold had been crushed by Avery Brundage and his cohorts at the IOC.

Years later, tests revealed Clarke had ruptured a small muscle in his heart, the one that controls the mitral valve that ensures the flow of blood in the heart will be pumped in the right direction. To say he had literally broken his heart in that 10,000 metre race, and all to no avail, is no exaggeration. Fortunately, he underwent a successful heart operation in Melbourne and was able to resume a normal life. The morning after his surgery he got out of bed and rode an exercise bike he had installed in his ward. A worried nursing sister asked his surgeon if it was all right for Clarke to be riding the exercise bike. 'I have no idea,' the doctor replied. 'I've never seen anyone do it before.'

I have to plead guilty to having missed the diagnosis of the ruptured mitral valve. My only defence is, at the time, no such injury had ever been reported anywhere in the world.

CZECH MATE

Ron Clarke did eventually get an Olympic gold medal. On a visit to Prague in what was then Czechoslovakia, he met up with Emil Zatopek, the great distance runner and four times Olympic champion, which included the unprecedented three gold medal successes in the 5000 metres, 10,000 metres and marathon at the 1952 Helsinki Games.

There is a lovely story told about Zatopek at Helsinki. After he successfully defended his 10,000-metre crown, his wife, Dana, won gold in the javelin. Emil was asked about running in the marathon, 'Right now the Zatopek family score is 2–1. That's too close for comfort. To restore prestige I think I must win the marathon.' The reporters then asked whether he would also run in the 5000 metres. He shrugged his shoulders and noted: 'The marathon won't be for a long while yet. In the meantime I need to do something.'

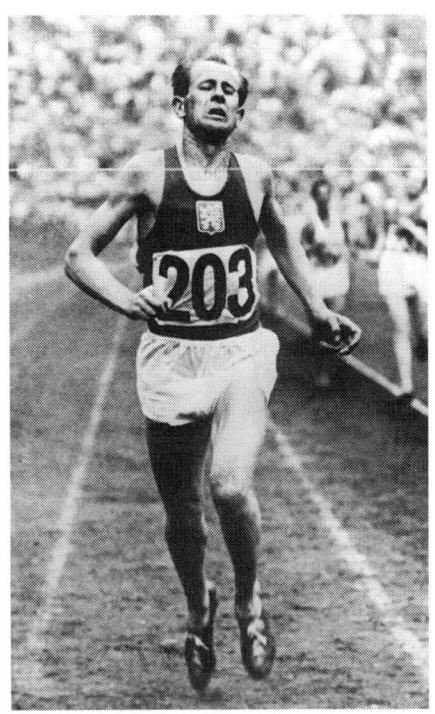

The extraordinary Czech athlete, Emil Zatopek, shown here winning the 1952 Olympic Marathon at Helsinki. (AAP IMAGE/AFP)

It was not ego, but a sense of fun.

Anyway, at the end of their meeting in Prague, Zatopek gave Clarke a small parcel.

'Don't open it until you are on the plane,' he ordered.

Clarke did as he was told. When he was airborne he opened the package and, to his amazement, there was one of Zatopek's gold medals, for the Helsinki 10,000-metre event. Zatopek had arranged for Clarke's name to be inscribed on it as well as his own.

It was a wonderful tribute from one great runner to another who undoubtedly deserved to have won an Olympic gold in his own right.

BY THE WAY, all our predictions given to the Australian Olympic Council before the Mexico City Games about the sprint and the track events in the rarified atmosphere proved spot-on.

The most dramatic illustration of this came in the long jump. The great Jesse Owens had been the first to top the 8 metre mark at the Olympics, leaping 8.06 metres at Berlin in 1936. This had stood as an Olympic record

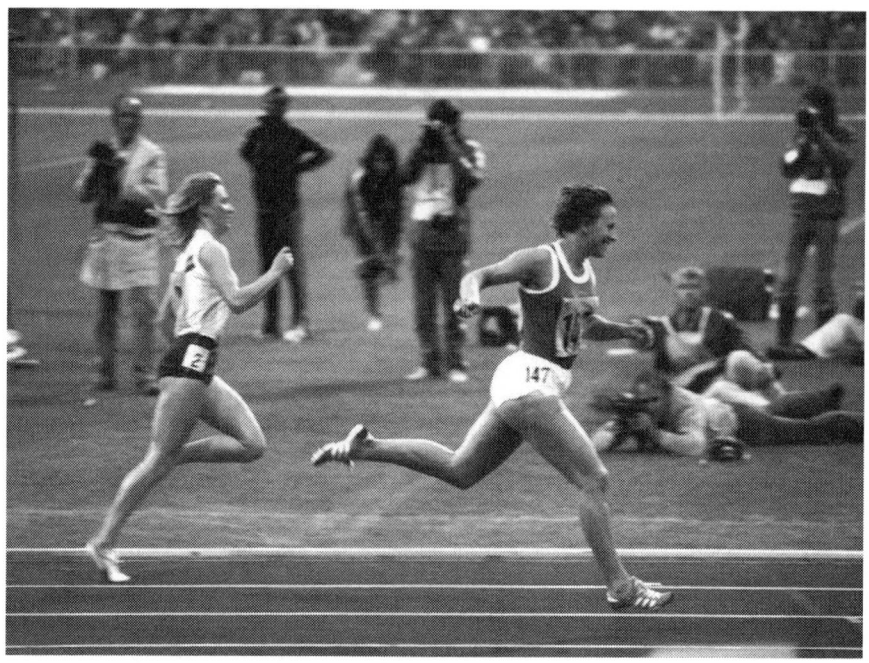

One of Australia's great athletes, Raelene Boyle, was beaten into second place in the 100 metres at the 1972 Munich Olympics by East German Renate Stecher.
(AAP IMAGE/SPORT THE LIBRARY/SPORTIMAGE/W. SCHULZE)

until a fellow American Ralph Boston jumped 8.12 metres at Rome in 1960. At Mexico City the first four competitors all beat the Olympic record. American Bob Beamon flew an incredible 8.90 metres to take the gold. Boston was in the competition but only managed third place. In the 33 years before Beamon's leap, the world record had improved by just 22 centimetres. In just a couple of seconds Beamon had advanced it by 55 centimetres. It just goes to show what a drop in air-pressure and resistance at altitude can do.

All was not doom and gloom for the Aussies at Mexico City. The 17-year-old Maureen Caird became one of the youngest ever Olympic athletics champions when she won the 80-metre hurdles from compatriot Pam Kilborn, the race favourite.

Another 17-year-old, Raelene Boyle, was a gutsy second to Poland's Irena Szewinska, who won the 200 metres in world record time. It was a great effort by Boyle against one of the greatest women athletes of all time: Szewinska (nee Kirszenstein) was the first athlete, male or female, to win a medal at four consecutive Olympics (1964–76).

Raelene seemed to have the world at her feet but was to suffer several disappointments at future Olympics. This was especially the case four years later in Munich when she was beaten into second place in both the 100 metres and 200 metres by East German Renate Stecher. In 1997, after the fall of the Berlin Wall, investigations into the obscene doping practises of the East German sporting coaches revealed that Stecher had been on a course of anabolic steroids for two years leading up to the Munich Olympics. Raelene was robbed of two gold medals by this drug cheat. But will the IOC hierarchy ever make amends to this wonderful Australian woman and give her the gold medals she so richly deserves? As the nineteenth century proverb explains — pigs might fly, but they are very unlikely birds.

Ralph Doubell, one of the athletes trained by Stampfl, surprised some of the general public by winning the 800 metres. Fellow Aussie Peter Norman, who had broken the world record when qualifying the previous day, split the American pair Tommie Smith and Juan Carlos to take silver in the final of the 200 metres. Smith and Carlos were sent home in disgrace at the behest of Avery Brundage after giving the Black Power salute while on the dais during the medal presentation. Norman,

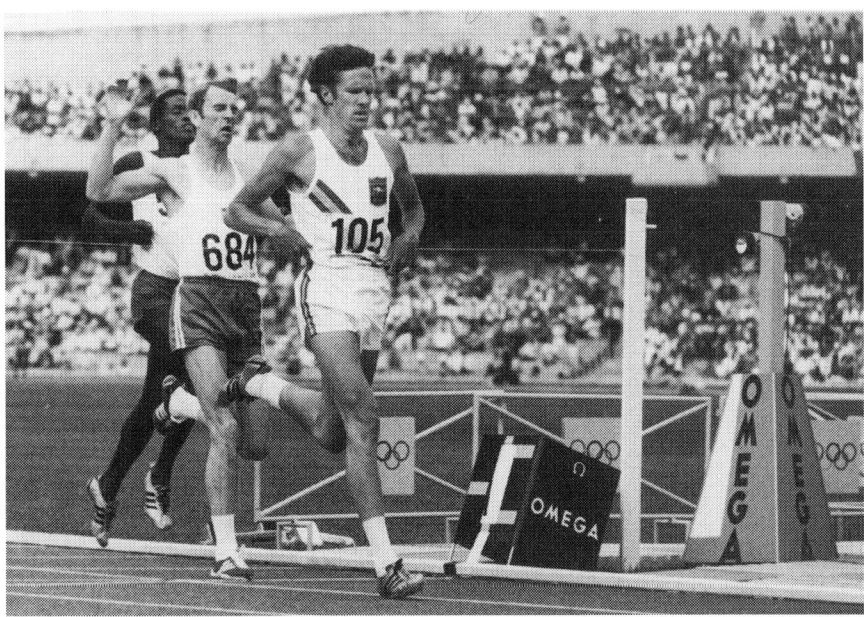

Ralph Doubell running in the 800 metres at Mexico, which he won.
(BRIAN CORRIGAN'S COLLECTION)

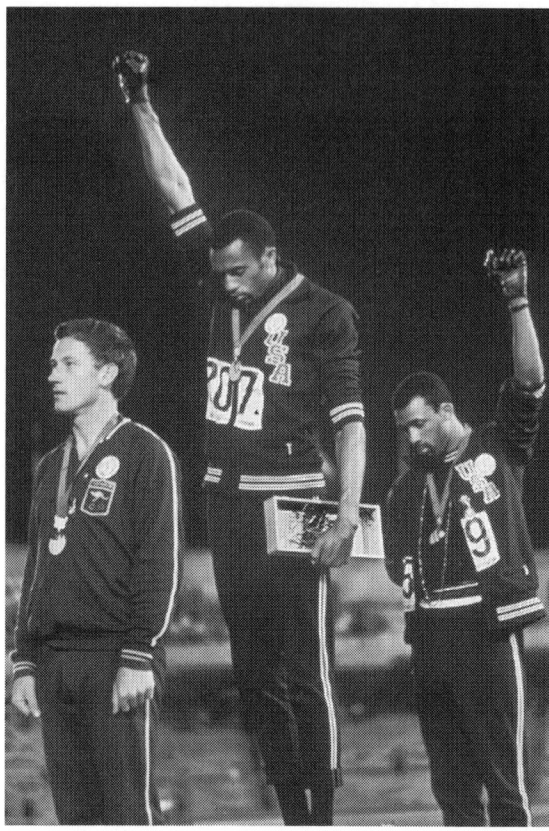

US athletes Tommie Smith (centre), winner of the 200 metres, and John Carlos (right) were sent home in disgrace because of their racial protest. Silver medallist Australian Peter Norman was reprimanded for wearing a civil rights badge in support. (AAP IMAGE/AP PHOTO)

a staunch Christian from a Salvation Army family, wore a civil rights badge given to him by the Americans. It was a brave stand.

IOC officials and many members of the media demanded Norman be treated the same as the Americans and sent home immediately. Our team leader Judy (Julius) Patching pulled Norman aside and his comments went something like this, 'I've been ordered to severely reprimand you. Consider that done. And by the way, I have some tickets for you for the hockey tonight.'

'Blood was spurting all over the arena as the matador fell lifeless to the ground.'

13. A GREAT IDEA

ONE OF THE problems for the athletes in Mexico City was boredom. By the end of the Olympics they would have spent six weeks in the city, and because of the security worries there was little for them to do, especially after they had completed their events.

I went to our genial Chef de Mission Judy Patching with some ideas. A first-rate people manager, Judy's Christian name was actually Julius — but no one had ever known him by any moniker other than Judy. Among the suggestions I had for overcoming the boredom was a visit to a bullfight.

'Great idea!' said Judy. 'Go ahead and organise it.'

Most of the athletes wanted to go and we were able to oganise some good seats right down the front of the *'sol y sombra'* section. This was one of the better areas to watch from — *sol* (sun) at the start, with *sombra* (shade) as it began to get really hot later in the day. Only a handful of the team had ever been to a bullfight, but the very idea of the colour, spectacle and music had everyone excited. They couldn't wait for the opening of the *corrida* (the fight).

The trumpets blasted. The crowd roared. And the first matador of the day strode out and proceeded to kneel on the ground, baring his bronzed chest, with his arms stretched wide as if to say to the bull, 'Here I am.' And there he was, the bull charged out of its corral. It ran, head down, straight at the matador. Indeed, straight into him. The bull's horns picked the matador up like a rag doll and tossed him high into the air. Blood was spurting all over the arena as the matador fell lifeless to the ground. It took just a moment, but he was D-E-A-D.

'Wow,' shouted one Aussie newspaperman. 'That was great! I caught every moment of it with my movie camera.' No doubt to show his young kids back home. There was no such enthusiasm among the members of the Australian Olympic team. I looked around. At first the blood drained from their faces. Then it was pandemonium. The girls were screaming. They were hysterical, not to mention the members of the swimming team. I had forgotten they were just kids.

The Mexicans in the crowd around us were not at all sympathetic, especially those whose view of the bloodshed was being obscured by the chaos that had engulfed the young Australian women. There was whistling and catcalls and cursing, and a shower of cushions rained down on the distraught Aussie girls. I didn't understand Spanish but it was obvious they were shouting for us to get lost, to get out of the arena and let them watch the next episode in the slaughter.

Many members of the team fainted. How do you get them out of the arena? Every available team official was pressed into service to carry them up the steep stairs to the outside. Too many of these officials were, shall we say, ancient. And carrying bodies was a difficult task for them at the best of times, let alone at the high altitude of Mexico City. These very same officials were the ones who had refused to accept our predictions of what happens in the thin atmosphere were finding out first hand how right we had been.

They quickly started to run out of oxygen. They looked as if they were about to have heart attacks. They turned a lighter shade of pale, blue even! And a number of them collapsed, further blocking the passageways to the exit out of the arena. There was more jeering and whistling and throwing of cushions as the next bullfight was underway and the crowd's view was again being obstructed by these stupid Australians.

As I struggled to get several of these pale, panting officials to their feet I could not resist asking them, 'What do you think of the problem of altitude now?' They did not have sufficient breath to reply. However, to their credit they did subsequently admit that the altitude at Mexico City did indeed present a serious problem.

It took a while to get all the athletes and officials back to the Village. As the stragglers struggled to their rooms, Judy called me aside.

'Can I see you for a minute, Brian.'

A GREAT IDEA | 101

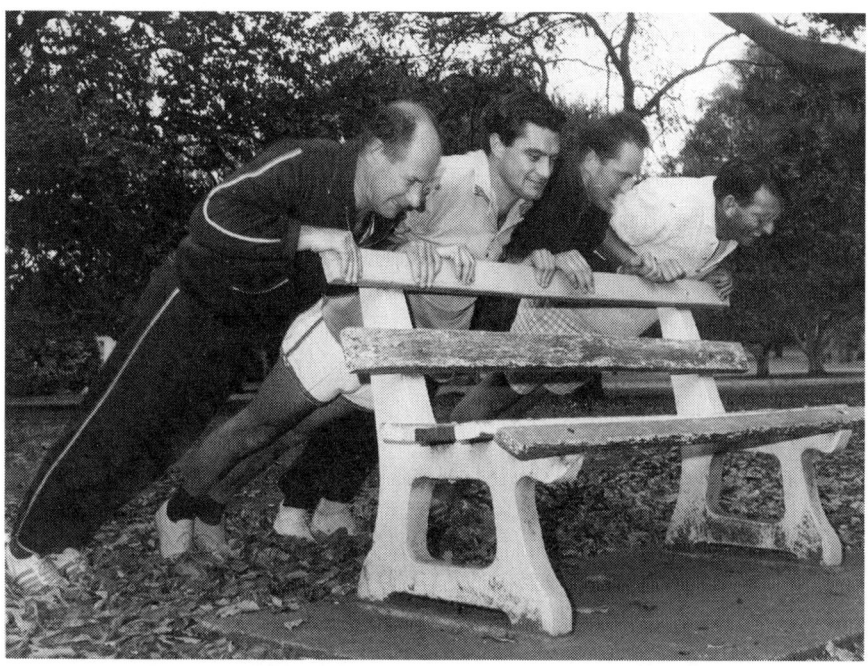

Good to see that even team officials take their fitness seriously: Julius 'Judy' Patching is on the left and I am suffering on the right, with David McKenzie and Bill Hoffman from the 1968 team in between. (BRIAN CORRIGAN'S COLLECTION)

'Certainly, Judy.'
'That was a great idea of yours.'
'Well thank you, Judy.'
'And you might do me a favour.'
'Certainly, Judy. What's that?'
'If you have any more bright ideas in the future, would you keep them to yourself?'
'Good idea, Judy!'

ONE EVENING TOWARDS the end of the Games, Judy Patching invited me to go with him to a most impressive dinner at which the guests included many of the IOC heavies. At the end of the night a couple of smooth young American men came up and after chatting for a while asked if I would like to accompany them in Howard Hughes' private plane on a trip to Acapulco the next day. Bring a friend, they said. So I asked Kerry O'Brien to come along. He had been unlucky enough just to miss out on a medal when only one second separated the first four place-getters in the 3000-metre steeplechase.

We were put up at the Las Brisas, the most opulent hotel in Acapulco at that time, where every room had its own private swimming pool and there was also the largest swimming pool with built-in bar I had ever seen. The Americans asked us what we would like to see first. That was easy; the famous divers who gracefully plummet between the 35 metre-high cliffs into the rock-strewn ocean below. The graceful swallow dives had a purpose. If they dive straight down they would be killed on the jagged rocks. So they have to dive outwards as well as down, a total distance of almost 42 metres. To avoid death they also have to time their dive for its conclusion to coincide exactly with the swell below carrying enough water with it. Of course, there had been some who had died, but we weren't going to be told how many.

The divers were resting in their hotel at this time of day, but that didn't deter our hosts who waved a fistfull of dollars in front of them and we had our own private viewing of this death-defying performance, including one spectacular effort when three of them dived at the same time.

After a sumptuous lunch, it was agreed we would all meet at the swimming pool at 5 p.m. 'Meanwhile, anything you want in Acapulco, anything at all, just let us know.' Both Kerry and I agreed there had to be some catch, but what was it?

We were sitting at the bar in the swimming pool right on five, when our two earnest young Americans appeared and swam out to join us.

'This is it,' I said.

There was no more mucking around.

'You know we represent Howard Hughes,' said the spokesman. 'He is interested in getting the Olympic Games for Los Angeles in 1976 and we want to know if he could have your vote.'

'My vote? I'm only the doctor for the Australian team!'

'Aw, hell, I thought you were the IOC delegate.'

As he swam off, he turned and shouted, 'Forget it. Just enjoy your stay.'

And without my vote Los Angeles did not get the Olympics for another 16 years. By that time Howard Hughes was dead. One of Hughes' associates was later implicated with a combined CIA–Mafia attempt to assassinate Cuban leader Fidel Castro. I felt sure I had met him that day.

SECOND OPINION

ALAN TRENGOVE

Respected Australian journalist and author. For 20 years Trengove was a feature writer and foreign correspondent for *The Herald & Weekly Times*. He has written many books including biographies of Prime Ministers Robert Menzies and John Gorton and sporting stars Ron Clarke, Herb Elliott, Keith Stackpole and Geoff Hunt, as well as the histories of BHP and the Davis Cup.

CONFIDENCE AND TRUST

I FIRST MET Brian at the bar of a pub in Pembrokeshire, South Wales in 1961. I was working in the London Bureau of *The Herald & Weekly Times* and covering the arrival of a large contingent of the German Army, which was going to train in Wales as part of a NATO exercise. With World War II still fresh in many memories, it was a quite controversial episode.

Brian was travelling with the Australian cricket team on an Ashes tour of Britain. One of my initial impressions was that you couldn't pick him as being a doctor. He actually looked indistinguishable from the players and generally conducted himself like one of the cricketers. He was about the same age as some team members and loved the game as much as they did, perhaps, in the case of some of the players, even more. I quickly discovered he had a great sense of humour, was very down to earth, and was quick to unmask hypocrisy.

He also had, and still has, that marvellous quality of treating the highest and lowest in the social pecking order equally. To put it another way: he could treat a char-lady like a duchess, and a duchess like a char-lady, and, in doing so, charm both.

Over the next three or four years in London, Brian and I met each other intermittently. We occasionally had a beer together and played a few games of squash. He was absolutely crazy about sport, especially cricket. And I think that enthusiasm was largely responsible for the rapport he established with most sportspeople he treated or

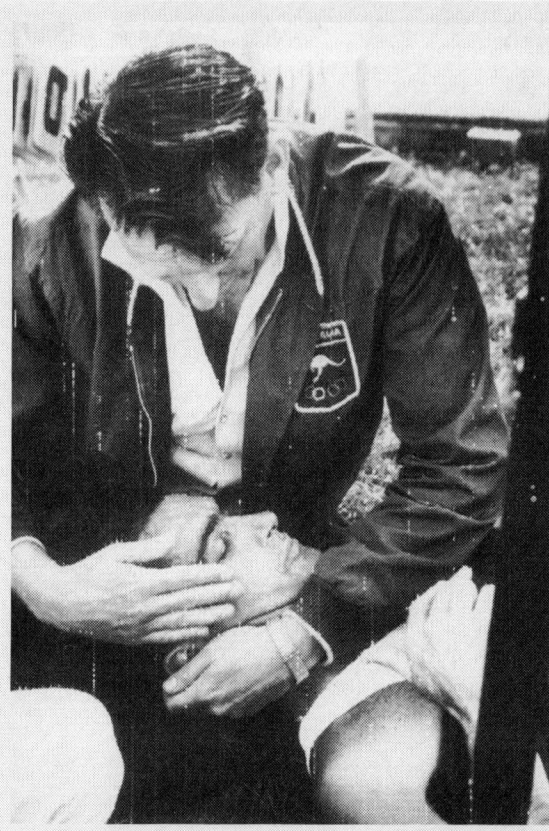

The image of me supporting Ron Clarke's head after he collapsed was sent around the world by the news wires. (BRIAN CORRIGAN'S COLLECTION)

came in contact with. I guess he instinctively understood the psyche of the elite sportsman and sportswoman.

In the context of the teams he was involved with, he was always very much a part of those teams. The champions and also-rans not only had the utmost faith in his medical ability, but valued his mateship and his genuine interest in their welfare.

A year or so ago I was with him at a Hall of Fame dinner in Melbourne when he bumped into Raelene Boyle. They hadn't seen each other for years and they hugged each other like affectionate family members. She was soon telling him uninhibitedly of the most dramatic moments of her more recent illnesses.

Ron Clarke is another champion who reveres him. I collaborated with Ron on his first book, an autobiography, and was at the Mexico City Olympics when he collapsed during the 10,000 metres from lack of oxygen in the thin atmosphere. The image of Brian kneeling over the prostrate Clarke in the middle of the arena, and burying his face in his hands and weeping at the misfortune that had befallen Clarke, is one of the most famous in Australian sport. It says, more than a thousand words of prose, and conveyed the warmth and compassion of Brian Corrigan. Somehow I managed to get into the van that took them back to the Olympic Village. They were both physically and mentally exhausted. I remember that they seemed to be in deep sleep, with Ron resting on Brian's shoulder, as we moved through the traffic.

IN ABOUT 1962, I bumped into Brian in Edinburgh. I was covering the Edinburgh Festival and he was then studying in the Scottish capital. I came to realise he was an extremely talented rheumatologist, though how he found the time to pursue his extended studies when he was so busy with his sports medicine tasks was a mystery. He had the knack of explaining medical complexities in layman's language, and was the very antithesis of the English concept of a staid and conservative member of the medical profession.

Later, he was a medical officer with the Arsenal football club in North London. That gave him the foundation for the many years of service he subsequently gave to Australian soccer. Arsenal was then, as it is now, one of England's premier soccer clubs. The fact that it chose Brian for medical advice was an impressive testimonial to his expertise.

BACK IN AUSTRALIA, we again met now and then, mainly when my work as a feature writer for the *Melbourne Sun* took me to Sydney. We collaborated on a book called *Living with Arthritis*, which took a practical approach to helping people understand the disease and guide them to useful strategies for overcoming its effects. Brian took a swipe at the quacks and charlatans who exploited people's misery and ignorance, ripping money off them with fake cures.

I remember being dismayed at Brian's workload. Trying to track him down was always a laborious business. He could be at any one of several hospitals, sometimes two or three in one day, or be at his practice in the northern Sydney beach suburb of Dee Why, or at some sports venue. I saw how he built confidence and trust in patients with his friendly beside manner. He often laid his hands on patients, reassuringly. Medicine was never a means of making a fortune. Quite the contrary! And every patient was an individual in whom he invested his own personal interest and care.

At the same time, he carried on his sports medicine interests with tremendous zest and, as far as I know, little or no monetary reward. He was one of the pioneers of sports medicine in Australia. In more recent years, he became one of this country's leading authorities on the illegal use of drugs in sport. His common sense, another of his outstanding traits, has advanced the fight to eradicate such abuse.

The world could do with many more like him. But that would not be possible. For there is no other like Brian Corrigan. He is unique!

> 'The morning after the horror a simple but incredibly moving remembrance ceremony was held in the main stadium, with 11 empty chairs for the dead Israelis serving as a heart-wrenching symbol.'

14. THE SHATTERED DREAM

THE OLYMPIC GAMES had been conceived as a way of bringing people together in peace, as a truce from world politics. Maybe they had never previously quite lived up to that image. But if it were a dream, it was a dream worth pursuing. And I, for one, believed in that dream.

The Munich Olympics in 1972 turned this dream into a nightmare, on a bleak, September day. That day the Games were stripped of their innocence and apolitical façade. The whole world, particularly the Olympic world, was so shattered that the Olympics could never be the same again.

After that we were besieged with problems of shamateurism, under-the-lap payments to athletes, television with its obscene amounts of money, political boycotts, drugs, cheating, the East German regime and its corruption.

The Munich Olympics will always be associated with the great tragedy that befell the Israeli team on 5 September when two athletes were killed and nine others were captured and held hostage by eight Palestinian terrorists. This was accompanied by a series of incredibly inept actions by the German authorities and police, who spent a day in negotiations with the terrorists as deadline after deadline passed. German police, obvious in tracksuits and carrying suspicious-looking bags, were everywhere. Late that night the terrorists bundled the nine hostages off to the Fuerstenfeldbruck Airport in the hope that they (the terrorists) could escape. The police ambushed them, resulting in the death of the nine hostages, five of the terrorists and one policeman.

BEFORE THE GAMES, the German authorities had announced that security would be incredibly tight, and there were a large number of security people running around. After the first few days or so, we found security to be all rather slack, even more so by the second week. There was no problem at all for visitors to get into the Village without a pass. Many visitors would just wear a tracksuit top and wave to the guards who would wave back.

Some officials in our team would go for an early morning run and, to get out from the back of the Village where we were, would scale a high fence and run around the Village perimeter. I'd be lagging behind since they could climb and run a lot faster, but I found a short cut where the perimeter fence was very low as it had a built-up mound of earth on one side of it that was really simple to climb. I used to do this most mornings to get back into the Village, and noticed other teams would use the low part of the fence too. The street I ran down was the very street where the Israeli quarters were located. It was all so easy for the terrorists.

The Games were suspended on the day of the massacre. The morning after the horror a simple but incredibly moving remembrance ceremony was held in the main stadium, with 11 empty chairs for the dead Israelis serving as a heart-wrenching symbol. The atmosphere was ruined by a most inept, unsympathetic political speech by IOC President Avery Brundage, who had insisted the Games would go on despite all that carnage. Life certainly was never the same after the tragedy.

I have often been asked which of the eight Olympics I have been involved with was my favourite. Had it not been for 5 September, I would definitely have said Munich. I suppose it might be a little like asking, 'And apart from that did you enjoy the play, Mrs Lincoln?' Before that day, the 1972 Munich Games had been, and would remain, the most felicitous and friendly of any sporting event I ever attended, made more so because of individuals with whom I was involved.

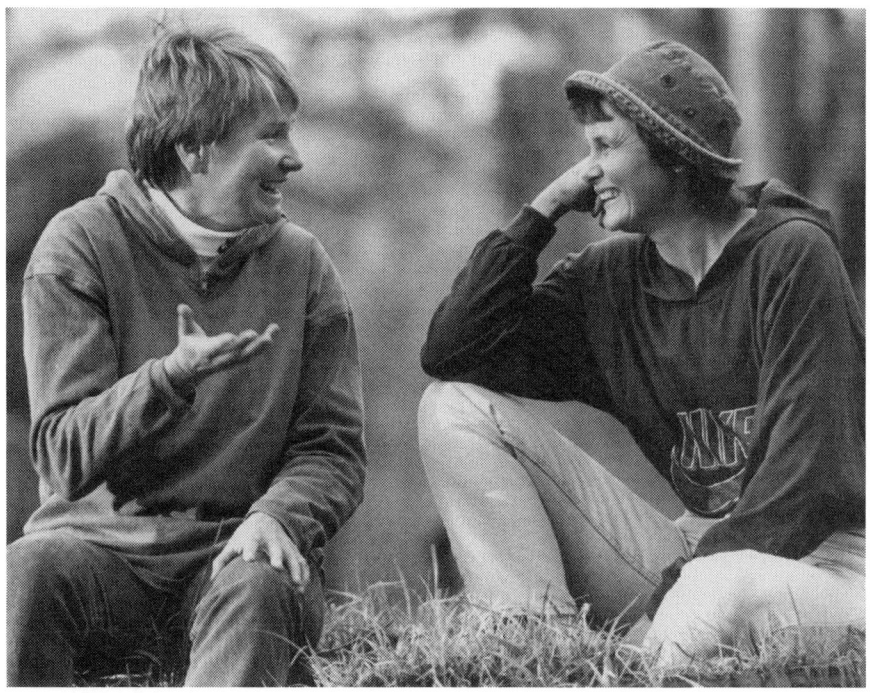

Two of Australia's most famous athletes from the 1972 Munich Olympics together again, twenty years later. Raelene Boyle (left) and Shane Gould.
(AAP IMAGE/SPORT THE LIBRARY)

OF COURSE, THE Munich Olympics was a triumph for teenager Shane Gould who won gold medals in the 200-metre and 400-metre freestyle and the 200-metre individual medley as well as a silver in the 800-metre freestyle and a bronze in 100-metre freestyle (see *Chapter 29 — Pros and Cons*). Had it not been for the incredible effort of American Mark Spitz in winning seven gold medals she would have been feted as the star of the Games. There were three other golds won by Australians in Munich, all by swimmers — Gail Neall (400-metre individual medley), Bev Whitfield (200-metre breaststroke); and Brad Cooper (400-metre freestyle). And the Aussie yachtsmen won two golds up at Kiel on the Baltic Sea, in the Dragon (John Cuneo, Tom Anderson and John Shaw) and Star (David Forbes and John Anderson). Indeed, the yachties provided history. The Brisbane twins John and Tom Anderson hold a unique place in the history of the Olympics, having won gold medals at the same Olympics, on the same day, at virtually the same time, but on different boats.

I HAVE SOME stark memories of the Munich Olympics, other than the terrorism tragedy. When one of our rowing coaches, Alan Callaway, suddenly started to vomit huge quantities of blood at three o'clock one morning, we had to get him to hospital as quickly as possible. I don't know if you have ever thought about how that could be organised in Germany in the dead of night, but finally we were able to contact an ambulance and arrange transport to the Krankenhaus, the local hospital. The ambulance driver's instructions were to drop us at the front door, which is exactly what he did. It was dark and cold and the huge hospital was a most forbidding sight.

We opened the door and, with not a soul in sight, walked along a long, dark, eerie Kafka-esque passageway. Alan was not feeling very well at all. No stretchers about, so nothing else to do but walk to the end and then up the flight of stairs to the next landing. There was not a soul in sight up there either. So it was then up to the next landing where at last we spied a light. It belonged to the nursing station, thank heavens. Sitting inside were two gay male nurses. I managed to explain to them, using my small amount of German and with their small amount of English, that I had a very sick man who needed urgent attention. They did not appear to be very concerned with our plight, although it turned out they had been expecting us.

We weren't making a great deal of headway until I saw a photo of the entertainer Shirley Abicair on the wall. She was very big in Europe at that time. Some readers may remember her for her expertise in playing the zither, the plucked musical instrument responsible for the haunting Harry Lime theme in the Orson Welles movie *The Third Man*. I was genuinely surprised to see her photo.

'Ah, Shirley Abicair,' I said, pointing at the photo. 'She is an Australian, too.' The pair was absolutely delighted to hear this.

'Oh, vee loff her,' they said, rolling their eyes in unison. 'She is wunderbar. You know her?' As if Australia was the size of Dresden!

'Of course,' I lied, I did at least have a good friend who knew her well. They couldn't do enough for us after that and fussed around Alan until he was tucked up in his hospital bed. They rang a taxi for me and I was able to get back to the Village.

I was then struck with serious doubts, worrying about what would happen to him. After all, no doctor had seen him by the time I left him. I was back at the hospital, which was now buzzing with activity, at eight o'clock next morning. Alan was sitting up in bed, a wide smile on his face and no longer wearing the deathly pallor of the previous night. I needn't have worried at all about his welfare. The doctor reported he had already had a blood transfusion and had had a camera inserted into his stomach to make sure the bleeding didn't re-occur. Alan was able to go home next morning. It could never have happened that fast in Australia at that time.

I should never have doubted the efficiency of German hospitals.

IT IS DIFFICULT to believe in these more enlightened times, but there was a time when males and females in the Olympic Village were segregated; separated by a high wire fence and guards. It was like that in Munich, and did not alter at the Olympics for many years.

Doctors were allowed to go into the female quarters with their pass, but, again, security had been pretty slack. After a while I got to know the guards and they would just wave as we went in to visit a patient.

The hurdler Penny Gillies suffered a nasty rearfoot fracture in competition and was confined to her room. On the day after the Israeli disaster, I was going to visit her and at the same time I was carrying a pair of trousers that I was taking to be dry-cleaned. By now security was completely different, soldiers with machine guns were stationed all around the compound. The entrance was guarded by a blonde German Amazon, in jackboots no less, and carrying a revolver in her holster. If she had had a whip she could have passed for one of the notorious guards during an infamous era 30 years before. In my mind, she went by the name of Ilsa Koch.

When I got to the gate, I told her who I was and why I was there.

'Vere is your pass?' she demanded.

Of course, I did not have it with me. 'Ilsa' waved her hand to dismiss me. There was a most definite 'Nein!' No way could I come in. Orders were orders. Just then, she was distracted by another doctor who had exactly the same problem, so I took my chance and bolted in. She was screaming at me in German, blowing her whistle and I thought at any moment she might even fire her revolver at me.

I made my way through the labyrinth of huts that sheltered the female athletes and had a look at how Penny was getting on (not very well, I should say). When I was leaving, I could see Ilsa, furious, waiting for me. I had almost reached the gate when I suddenly remembered. I had left my dry-cleaning behind. What else to do but turn around and make another race to get inside. That really caused a commotion, but I grabbed my trousers as quickly as I could, and returned to face the music. It wasn't music; it was a torrent of abuse.

'Vere is your pass?'

'I have already told you that I do not have it on me,' was the honest answer.

'So vot iss your name, I will see to it that you vill be expelled from the Village.' And there was not doubt she believed she could arrange such an expulsion.

'Julius L Patching.' And she carefully wrote it down. I departed, her eyes burning a hole through the back of my head, dropped off my dry-cleaning and headed back to our headquarters. I thought it would be much easier to be abused by Judy Patching than by her. Besides, he had far more pressing problems on that day than having to worry about his errant doctor.

SECOND OPINION

RAELENE BOYLE

One of the greatest sprinters in the history of Australian athletics. Winner of three Olympic silver medals (in 1968 and 1972), having been robbed of two golds by East German drug cheat Renate Stecher in the 1972 Games.

ABSOLUTE INSPIRATION

WHEN YOU NORMALLY think of doctors you conjure up visions, probably quite unfairly, of conservative types with little sense of humour. Brian Corrigan never fitted that description. He was quite the opposite, a larrikin type of doctor who slotted so well into an Olympic team. Not there to order you around, but would try to make you feel relaxed, feel at home, and be fit and ready to perform at the highest level.

I was only a kid when I first met him on the plane en route to the 1968 Mexico Olympics. He and Howard Toyne were the team doctors. I knew Howard because he was from Melbourne, but it was my initial encounter with Brian and I soon realised he was not your 'normal' type of doctor.

The pair of them looked after me on my first great adventure. I was so homesick and after about two weeks I wanted to go home. To try to make me feel part of the family they decided to take me on an outing, sampling the culture of Mexico City. It was a real eye opener. There was a training school for Andalusian dancing horses near the village. That was our first stop-off and the memories of those wonderful horses remain in my memory. There were also a few sights that weren't so wonderful, including some cock fighting that attracted a big crowd of locals. Being a young animal-loving girl from Coburg I felt quite ill, but the doctors were showing me how people from the other side of the world spent their lives, introducing me to the real world.

Doc Corrigan became a true friend at those Olympics, nursing the injuries of both my body and brain, nurturing this youngster through what was an extraordinary event. The doctors didn't have fixed ideas about how one should live life. There was no 'That's right' or 'That's wrong'. For example, I used to enjoy a beer (and still do), particularly before I went to bed. It helped relax me. The docs talked to the team bosses to ensure I was allowed those beers.

DOC CORRIGAN BECAME a real inspiration later in my life by the way he fought his cancer. He was a very sick man when he went into the operation to remove the brain tumour (see *Chapter 33 — A Brain Tumour*). How did he cope? He succeeded because of an incredibly positive attitude to life. The cancer was not going to beat him. No way!

When I was also forced to face cancer some years later, I thought of the way he reacted. It was at the forefront of my mind, if people like him could get over it, win the battle, so could I.

A wonderful guy — an absolute inspiration!

'The first question went something like: "Why were you such a failure?" A failure? He [Steve Holland] had just swum his heart out to break the world record, for Gawd's sake.'

15. PRIME MINISTER BOOED

THE 1976 MONTREAL Olympics was a financial disaster. There was a massive blow-out in the building costs, which had threatened to send the city bankrupt. The hard-hit citizens of Montreal contemptuously dubbed the Olympics 'The Big Owe'. The debt was so big that it was not paid off until recently.

Problems involving the lack of planning, corruption and alleged money laundering by the Mafia threatened to cancel the Games. On the day of the Opening Ceremony, workmen could be seen still trying to finish the Stadium. It actually was not finally finished until some years later.

There was also, for that time, the inevitable political argument over South Africa and apartheid. Sixteen African nations, with Tanzanian president Julius Nyerere as their spokesman, threatened a boycott because the New Zealand Rugby Union All-Blacks had toured South Africa. The fact that South Africa was already banned from the Games mattered not. The Africans wanted the New Zealand team expelled from the Olympics too. The 16 protesting nations sent their teams to Montreal to increase the pressure. The IOC ruled, quite correctly, that Rugby was not one of their sports so they had no jurisdiction. The Olympic chiefs stood firm against all the pressure and the 16 African nations, as well as Iraq and Guyana, walked out. Guyanese sprinter James Gilkes asked to be allowed to compete as an individual, but the IOC ruled athletes must compete for their countries and rejected his plea.

The other political argument was the problem of the conflict between China and Taiwan over which country should legitimately be representing China. The Canadian Prime Minister, Pierre Trudeau, under immense pressure from China, which was the largest buyer of Canadian wheat, had refused entry for the Taiwanese unless they agreed to march under the Olympic banner and not under their own flag. The IOC blasted the decision as political interference and in the end Trudeau had to relent. As a result, China withdrew its team from the Games and had to wait another day before making its Olympic debut.

MY INVOLVEMENT IN the Montreal Olympics came about entirely by chance when I ran into an old friend, Les Mills, in Sydney. Les and his wife, Colleen, were outstanding sportspeople, both having represented New Zealand in athletics, Les in the shot put and discus, Colleen as a sprinter. (Les was later to become Mayor of Auckland and set up a successful chain of gymnasiums across New Zealand.) He had a deep knowledge of sport and sport training methods and had just finished as Papua New Guinea's (PNG) coaching director, where he had made a huge contribution by setting up clinics and facilities. Les was appointed adviser to the PNG team for the Montreal Games. He asked if I would like to go as their medical officer and I jumped at the chance. It was only a small team, lacking in experience and overwhelmed by the big city atmosphere. In fact, the marathon runner was so overwhelmed that he went 'bush' for a few days. Their two boxers took a terrible hiding.

Australia's 1976 Olympic team did poorly. It was a great disappointment after its big success in Munich, and provided a great shock to the athletes and to the Australian public at large. The Aussies finished with just one silver medal and four bronze. Not since Berlin in 1936 had an Australian team failed to finish an Olympics without at least one gold medal. It was as if the rest of the world was going forward, while Australia was going backwards.

One problem was the lack of facilities and sponsorship due to a lack of government interest and funding. Things weren't improved when the Prime Minister, Malcolm Fraser, turned up in the Village, as so many politicians do, for his press photo opportunity with the Olympic team and the athletes loudly booed him and called him many nasty names. He had never shown any interest in them or their funding difficulties before, and they weren't going to fall all over him for the cameras now.

Some good did finally come out of the team's display in Montreal. The Federal Government was forced into doing something about the funding problem, which lead to the creation of the well-financed and world-renowned Australian Institute of Sport (AIS).

WHEN AUSTRALIA PLAYED New Zealand in the Montreal hockey final, I saw one of the most courageous performances imaginable. Late in the game, with New Zealand holding on to a 1–0 lead, the Kiwi goalkeeper, Trevor Manning, was hit a sickening blow (from Ric Charlesworth, if my memory serves me correctly) which shattered his kneecap. He should have gone off, anyone else would have. Manning opted to stay on. In the final few minutes, from a few metres out a smash from Ian Cooke came in, seemingly for a certain goal that would tie it up for Australia. Manning stuck his fractured kneecap in the way to foil the Aussies' chances. Unbelievable! There is no way in the world I could have done that. He didn't walk properly for a long time afterwards and to this day has a piece of wire in his knee holding it together. New Zealand owed the 1–0 gold medal victory to the courage that day of Trevor Manning.

The 1500-metre freestyle swim was a great race with the Australian Steve Holland involved. He was a brilliant swimmer and the reigning world champion. He had also held the world record for that distance, on and off, over the previous three years, although American Bruce Goodell had recently beaten it. Since no Aussie had won a gold medal at Montreal it seemed all Australia including the media was determined this would be the big chance. Steve just couldn't lose. His problem was he had the two American stars, Goodell and Bobby Hackett in the same race. They swam a brilliant tactical race to finish first and second, both going under the existing world record. Holland also broke the world record by two seconds to finish third.

The media that had hyped him so much before this event now turned against him. Most typical was the interview by one Sydney television commentator. The first question in the interview went something like: 'Steve, why were you such a failure?' A failure? He had

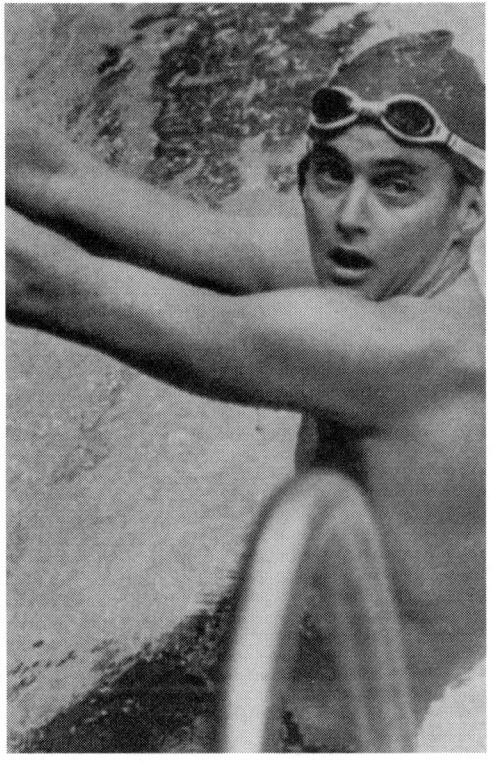

Steve Holland, training for the 1976 Montreal Olympics. The Australian media's response to his superb bronze medal in the 1500-metre freestyle, in which he broke the world record, was so dispiriting that he retired from swimming soon after. (AAP IMAGE/SPORT THE LIBRARY)

just swum his heart out to break the world record, for Gawd's sake. Steve just stared and had difficulty in answering that one.

Soon after the race Steve received a call from Malcolm Fraser to offer his congratulations. This made Steve really mad because money had been particularly tight and Fraser had never done a thing to help. He said something along the lines of, 'Mate, where were you when I needed you and I wouldn't vote for you, so get lost.' Holland later swam in the 400-metre freestyle final, but his heart did not seem in it. He finished fifth in the race which was also won by Goodell. Soon after the Games, a disillusioned Steve Holland retired from swimming.

Australia's three other medals at Montreal were bronze. The equestrian team was third in the three-day event and Australia finished third in both the Finn and 470 class yachting.

The hard-luck story of Australia's performance at the Montreal Olympics was sprinter Raelene Boyle. Boyle carried the Australian flag at the Opening Ceremony. She was the first woman given that honour, and there could not have been a more deserving person, especially as it has since been discovered that she had been cheated out of gold medals at Munich four years earlier by an East German drug cheat. Raelene was among the favourites to win gold in the 100 metres and 200 metres at Montreal. In the 100 metres she finished a close fourth in the final after a very slow start. She had been forced to dwell at the blocks because of being called for a false start earlier.

Disaster struck in the 200 metres. It was Boyle's favourite event, one in which she had finished second at the previous two Olympics. Sadly in the semi-final she was disqualified for two false starts. The first time she had not left the blocks early, but the starter claimed she had moved her head and shoulders as he fired the gun (a judgment shown to be incorrect by the television coverage). Unsettled by the incredible decision Boyle unbelievably left the blocks before the gun had sounded in the restart and was out of the event. Disqualified.

Raelene never won that Olympic gold she so richly deserved. Like that other great Australian sprinter, Betty Cuthbert, Raelene moved up to the 400 metres and was chosen for the team to go to the 1980 Moscow Olympics. The bitter debate about whether athletes should boycott the Moscow Games proved too much and Raelene decided to stay at home. She finished her running career in a blaze of glory at the age of 31, winning the 400 metres at the Brisbane Commonwealth Games.

CRICKET ... TRAGIC

The booing of Prime Minister Malcolm Fraser by members of the 1976 Olympic team was not surprising. After all, Fraser was always uncomfortable around sporting people, especially those from working-class backgrounds.

A story, possibly doubtful, is told of Fraser that soon after the Montreal Olympics he was advised to change his unpopular image by appearing to be interested in sport.

'Very well,' he replied to his advisor. 'What do you suggest?'

The West Indian cricket team was playing in Brisbane at the time and Fraser agreed, as part of this new image, to meet the Windies' captain, Viv Richards, and his Australian counterpart, Greg Chappell. When they were brought to meet him, the new sports lover is said to have asked, 'Now, which of you is Viv Richards?'

'On more that one occasion the Soviets were accused, and with very good reason, of cheating.'

16. RUSSIAN ROULETTE

THE OLYMPIC GAMES held in Moscow in 1980 were highly controversial as they were subject to more political pressure than any other. It seemed the whole world, even down to families and friends, was divided. In 1978, a military coup in Afghanistan installed a pro-Soviet regime. Over the following 12 months this regime battled Muslim guerrillas and became increasingly reliant on the USSR. In the last days of 1979 Soviet combat troops were airlifted into Afghanistan to help prop up the regime. By the end of January 1980, some 85,000 Soviet troops were operating inside the country even though the Soviet invasion was publicly denied by Soviet leader Leonid Brezhnev. The United States imposed sanctions on the Soviet Union and President Jimmy Carter called for a worldwide boycott of the Games ordering the American team to stay at home. He actually threatened to revoke the passport of any athlete who defied the ban and went to Moscow. It was an election year, but that wouldn't have influenced him though, would it? Ironically, as it turned out, one of the major reasons for the eventual fall of communism in the Soviet Union and its Iron Curtain allies was the Soviet involvement in Afghanistan.

In Australia, the coalition government of Malcolm Fraser fell over itself in its speed to support Carter's Olympic stand, putting immense pressure on the independent Australian Olympic chiefs to agree to a boycott. The Australian Olympic Federation (AOF) was unwilling to bow to the political pressure for several reasons, not least because Australia was one of only a handful of countries to have been to every one of the modern Olympics. The AOF vote to go ended up extremely close, just a single vote, seven to six, but it defied the Federal Government and we were on our way.

Several sports, for example, the men's and women's hockey teams decided not to go. Others had succumbed to the Fraser government's offer of a bribe, although it was never, of course, called that — it was 'financial assistance'. The athletes of those sports that did decide to compete all had the right to vote on whether they would go or stay at home. Some athletes didn't go to Moscow because they had genuine doubts, and this was respected. In the end, there were more who went (190 athletes and officials) than those who stayed at home (about 80).

IT WAS A gala day in Moscow for the Opening Ceremony. At the march-in, 81 countries were represented. The flags of 16 countries, including Australia, were not carried. Instead, as a sign of protest, the Olympic flag was used. Russian television did not show those 16 Olympic flags, only the flags of the USSR and countries that supported them. It's called censorship. Australian Chef de Mission, Phil Coles, made a clever move when, in a gesture of unity, he decided the flag would be carried by a male and a female, swimmer Max Metzker and athlete Denise Boyd. An Olympic first.

Moscow at night is surprisingly beautiful with the Red Square and the Kremlin brilliantly lit. Its wide streets were amazingly empty. All the school children had been sent away to the country and the derelicts rounded up. Virtually the only transport to be seen on the streets were large black Government cars with windows covered so no one could see in, rushing along in some small convoy in or out of the Kremlin. That emptiness is even more incredible when contrasted with the massive, barely moving Moscow traffic jams of today.

The Games themselves went off peacefully enough, with huge security in place, and the Russians kept making a great deal out of their so-called Solidarity and Friendship. Such shibboleths flew out the Lenin stadium when the Games began. On more than one occasion the Soviets were accused, and with very good reason, of cheating. One was when a gate in the Lenin stadium was 'accidentally' left open for a time, allowing their javelin thrower to benefit from the stiff breeze through the tunnel.

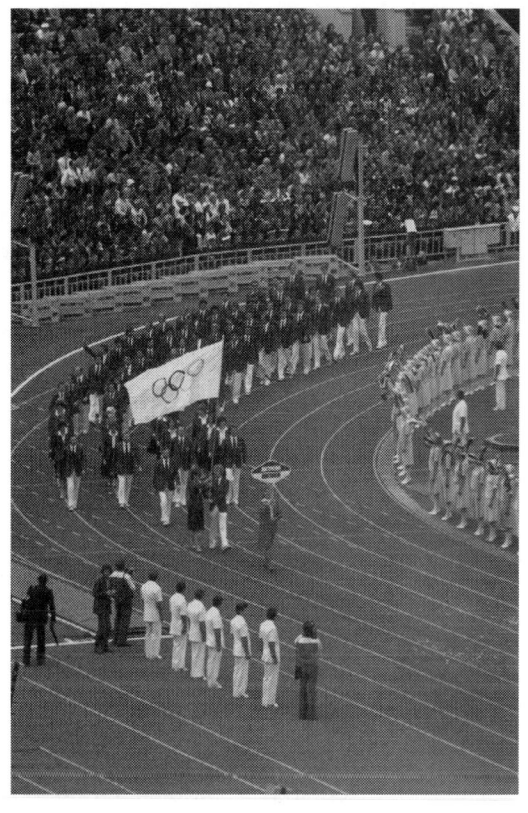

High controversy attended the 1980 Moscow Olympics. A number of countries did not send teams, supporting a US boycott. Australia did in the end go but chose not to carry the Australian flag at the opening ceremony, instead marching under the Olympic banner held by Max Metzker and Denise Boyd.
(AAP IMAGE/SPORT THE LIBRARY/PRESSE SPORTS)

Another such 'incident' happened in the triple jump (the old hop, skip and jump). The Soviet judges seemed intent on trying to ensure that Russian Viktor Saneyev would go into the history books as the second athlete to win four consecutive gold medals. Australian Ian Campbell and world record holder, Joao Carlos de Oliveira of Brazil, had a host of questionable decisions go against them. Between them, the pair was charged with committing nine fouls in 12 leaps, an abnormally high number by such expert jumpers. Both athletes registered jumps which should have won the gold medal, only to see Soviet judges rule against them. Campbell's fourth jump was long enough to win the gold, but a judge claimed a foul. Campbell protested, but before any action could be taken, the sand in the pit was raked leaving no evidence of where he had landed. It was futile to take the matter further and Campbell, who had thrown in his job to train for the Moscow Games, had to be content with fifth place, with a leap well below his best. De Oliveira's final leap was well past that of the eventual gold medal winner, Jaak Uudmae of the

Soviet Union, but it, too, was deemed to be a foul. As it turned out, Saneyev wasn't good enough to win the event a fourth time and had to be content with the silver medal ahead of de Oliveira.

A NOTICEABLE FEATURE at first was the lack of atmosphere in the vast arenas because the number of spectators was so small. After a few days, the events suddenly became crowded. My cynical friend and colleague, Dr Brian Sando, suggested that this Russian version of rent-a-crowd came in two varieties according to how many roubles they received. The more poorly paid were only required to appear mildly interested at best, and sat glumly, looking bored, sometimes even with their back to the events. The better paid were enthusiastic and cheered, although only for the Soviet athletes of course.

This led to some nasty and unsporting incidents in several events, especially the pole vault. This had been an American preserve until 1972 when East German Wolfgang Nordwig won, followed in 1976 by Poland's Tadeusz Slusarski. The Moscow crowd would create an incredible din whenever a non-Russian was jumping, but seemed to reserve the greatest racket for the two Poles, Tadeusz Slusarski and Wladyslaw Kozakiewicz. Polish supporters in the stands responded in kind when the local athletes jumped. Despite the racket, the two Polish jumpers remained amazingly calm with Kozakiewicz finishing first and Slusarski second. They both made very rude, but the most expressive gestures towards the Russian crowd, letting them know what they thought of them. The Poles in the crowd responded by singing their old national anthem from pre-communist days. Kozakiewicz later provided the ultimate defiance of the communist way of life by defecting to West Germany.

Another scandal in the same event occurred when Sergei Kulibaba from Kazakhstan was found to be illegally giving directions about the wind conditions to his Soviet team-mate, Vladislav Volkov, who eventually finished third behind the two Poles. I wonder what Baron Pierre de Coubertin, the architect of the modern Olympics, would have made of all this.

AUSTRALIA WON TWO gold medals at Moscow, both in the swimming. The victory of the Australian team in the 4 x 100-metre medley relay

(Neil Brooks, Mark Kerry, Peter Evans and Mark Tonelli) became a part of Australian folklore because of the description of their efforts by the Australian Broadcasting Corporation (ABC) caller Norman May. As freestyler Brooks approached the finish, May was shouting into his microphone: '… five metres, four, three, two, one … Gold, Gold to Australia, Gold!' Most people remember the scream as just 'Gold, Gold, Gold!'

Michelle Ford made the most of the absence of fellow Australian Tracey Wickham, who had decided not to go to Moscow, by winning the 800-metre freestyle. Ford also won a bronze medal in the 200-metre butterfly. The East Germans, Ines Geissler and Sybille Schoenrock, finished 1–2 after they swam a team race designed to block Ford out of the gold medal. There were four other swimming bronzes: Graeme Brewer (200-metre freestyle); Metzker (1500-metre freestyle); Mark Kerry (200-metre backstroke); and Peter Evans (100-metre breaststroke). On the athletics track Victorian Rick Mitchell finished second in the 400 metres to a virtually unknown Soviet runner, Viktor Markin. And John Sumegi finished second in the 500-metre kayak singles (K1), the first time an Australian canoeist had won a medal in an individual event.

SOON AFTER OUR arrival in Moscow, my great friend and esteemed medical colleague, Ken Fitch, and I called into the Village Medical Centre to pay our respects to the Russian doctors, who arranged a meeting for 10 a.m. the next day. At this meeting Ken and I were seated on one side of a long table, with four of the Russian doctors on the other. It was a most desultory chat and our mouths were getting as dry as the conversation, but all they had to drink was some lukewarm, insipid orange-flavoured liquid. After more than an hour of this, the meeting broke up and then without a word, the table was loaded with vodka bottles. Things were certainly looking up! We toasted the health of everyone from their President Brezhnev to our Prime Minister Fraser and to the success of their medical team. We went on to make pretty little speeches swearing everlasting friendship.

I had never drunk vodka in my life before that, but it didn't seem to me to have too much of a bite, and the Russian doctors certainly were not showing any signs of wear. When it came time to stand up a very strange thing happened. I suddenly had great difficulty walking,

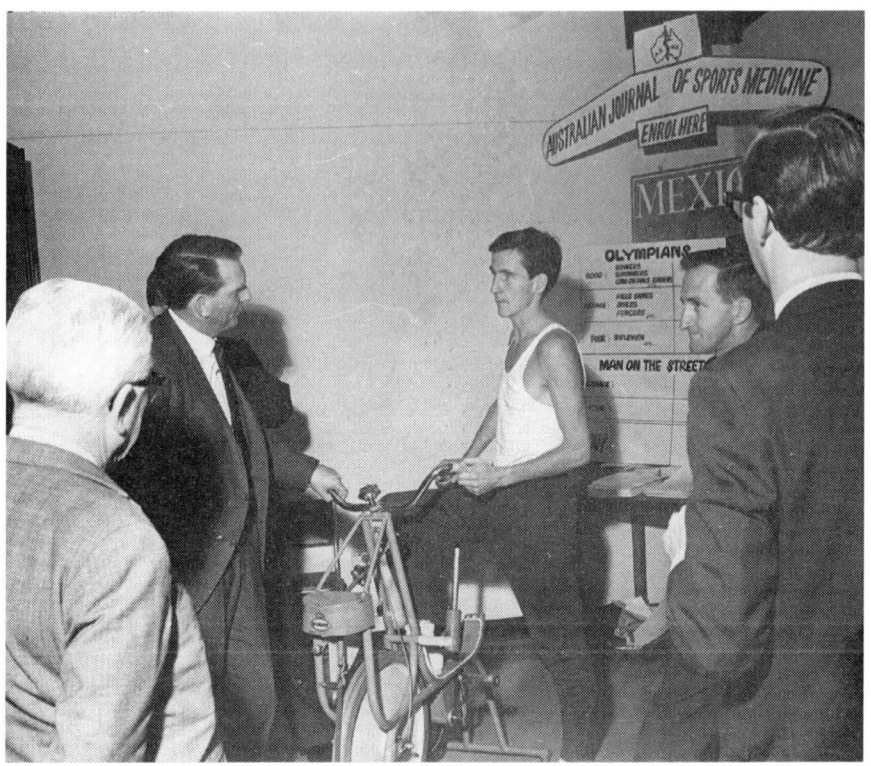

Testing Olympic Marathon runner John Farrington (centre) on a bicycle ergometer, with Ken Fitch on the right. (BRIAN CORRIGAN'S COLLECTION)

managing at least to get back home to get to bed for the rest of the day. That was the last time in my life I have ever drunk vodka.

The Russian doctors became good friends and would come to visit us, although I was never game to drink any more alcohol with them. They also invited us to visit their Polyclinic, the official athletes' clinic. They were so proud of the new equipment there. To our eyes all the equipment was shockingly antiquated, with an X-ray machine that was at least 40 years old and leaked radiation.

One night they rang us at our headquarters to ask if they could come around straightaway for a drink. This was a bit unusual as they usually arranged an appointment first. The doctors arrived looking absolutely dreadful.

'We have had the most terrible day,' their leader, Lev, told us. It transpired that an Irish newspaper had published an article that morning saying there was an epidemic of dysentery in the Village. It did seem most unlikely that it could be true for anyone to have this particularly nasty disease with its overtones of poverty, widespread plague-like contagion and death. The hierarchy at the Ministry of Health had rung them, furious and embarrassed, demanding they come up with an explanation on how to stop it.

The Irish team had their quarters right next to ours, so I asked the doctors to hang on for a minute and I would go and check with the Irish doctor. It turned out that at their morning press conference the Irish Chef de Mission was asked by a reporter if there were any health problems in the team.

'No, nothing much,' he replied.

'Are you sure you can't think of anything at all I could write about,' pleaded the reporter.

'Well, maybe a few cases of diarrhoea.'

'How do you spell that?' asked the pressman.

'Faith, I wouldn't know. You can just say dysentery, that's easier.'

That's how the Irish newspapers came to report the epidemic sweeping through the Olympic Village.

I MUST SAY I really didn't enjoy Moscow. The Russians we met in the Village were friendly and happy to talk as most spoke English, but outside the Village it was impossible to communicate with anyone and the bureaucracy was overbearing … quite stifling. Just one small example: we were invited to a dinner one night at the gigantic Cosmos Hotel. The passes we had were not sufficient to get us through the door. 'Nyet!' Special passes had to be issued. Where do you get them? At a place about a kilometre away. We got there. The man on duty was not the man who could issue them, we would have to wait until the proper official returned. We patiently waited. At last we had the proper piece of paper, walked back to the entrance of the hotel and the man at the door spent an age examining it. Once again, 'Nyet!' There was still something wrong with the pass. We would have to go back again. Stuff that … We left. Apparently many others had the same thought. On the flight home, via Vienna, an amazing thing happened. When the Captain announced that the aeroplane had just left Soviet airspace the whole planeload of athletes and officials from many countries stood up and cheered.

I had never seen anything like that before. I have never seen it since!

'Some members of the Australian boxing team took a marked dislike to one of their officials. So they ... bought a rat and a snake and tossed them into his room.'

17. HIGHS AND LOWS

IN 1984, THE Soviet Union and its Iron Curtain allies provided the payback to the Americans for their Moscow boycott by finding excuses not to attend the Olympics in Los Angeles. The Americans were unperturbed. They took the attitude that this merely meant more medals for them. Despite the absence of the Soviet bloc, the Los Angeles Olympics were quite successful with a record 140 nations taking part. They were also a commercial success returning a $US223 million profit. This financial triumph provided a model for future Olympics.

My involvement as doctor was mainly with the women's hockey team. It was the first real Olympic hockey tournament for the women. At Moscow, the first ever to be scheduled, five of the six nations who had qualified (all except the Soviet Union) took part in the boycott. The Moscow organisers had to rush around at the eleventh hour to find replacements. The team from Zimbabwe was only chosen the weekend before the Games and ended up winning gold.

Now, Australia had its chance. They first toured Germany, England and Vancouver. They had a skilful and determined team, well-managed and coached, and had high hopes for a medal, even gold, in the first past the post contest. They were bitterly disappointed at losing at the final hurdle. Coming into their last match against The Netherlands a win would have given them the gold medal. A one goal loss or a draw would have clinched the silver. But the Australians went down 2–0.

They were eventually placed fourth after a losing penalty shoot-out with the United States for the bronze medal. They made up for it four years later when they finally won their gold medal, as they also did in the Olympics at Atlanta in 1996 and Sydney in 2000.

The Los Angeles Games were one of the most successful of all time for Australia, with sportsmen and women winning 24 medals, including four golds. Only on home soil, at Melbourne in 1956, had an Australian team won more medals. The four golds went to heptathlete Glynis Nunn, weightlifter Dean Lukin and butterfly swimmer Jon Sieben, as well as the 4000-metre pursuit cycling team (Kevin Nichols, Michael Grenda, Michael Turtur and Dean Woods). To celebrate her success all Glynis wanted was a pavlova. Now finding a pavlova in Australia is pretty straightforward (after all we reckon we invented the dish). But in LA? Finding a pavlova in the city of angels proved more difficult than winning any gold medal. But we did it.

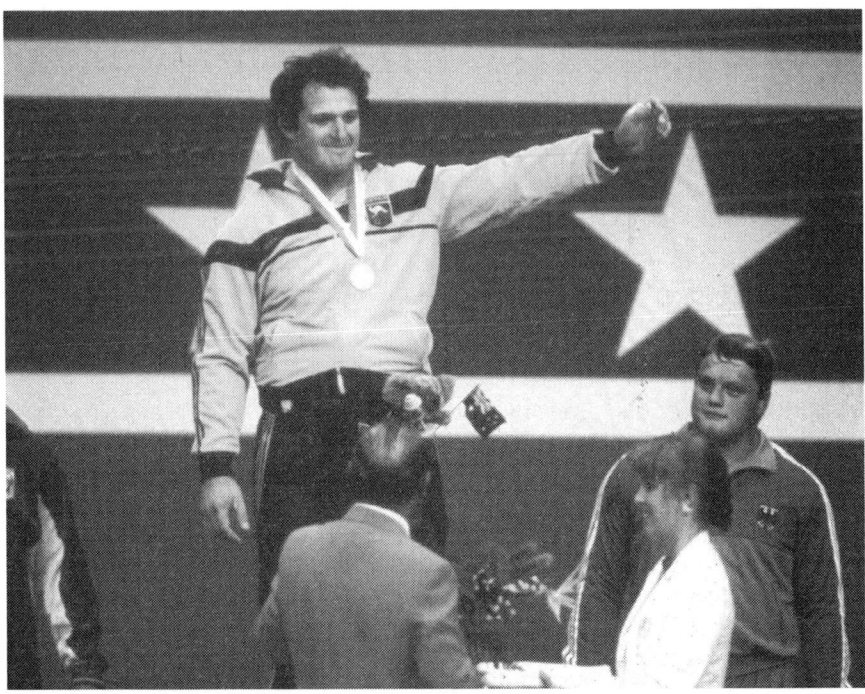

A gold-medal winner at one of Australia's most successful Olympic Games: Dean Lukin receives the gold for the super heavyweight weightlifting division at the 1984 Los Angeles Olympics. (AAP IMAGE/SPORT THE LIBRARY/ANDY HAYT)

Sieben, a Brisbane teenager was responsible for one of the greatest upsets in Olympic swimming history when he won the gold medal in the 200m butterfly. He beat two world record holders, West Germany's Michael Gross and American Pablo Morales, stopping the former from winning his third LA gold medal. Not only that, Sieben set a new world record of 1minute 57.04 seconds — which was more than four seconds faster than he had ever swum before going to Los Angeles. An incredible effort! Equestrian star Wayne Roycroft was Australia's flag-bearer at the Opening Ceremony, emulating his father, Bill, who had carried the flag at the 1968 Mexico City Olympics.

There was one offbeat incident at these Games. Some members of the Australian boxing team took a marked dislike to one of their officials. So they went out to a pet shop, bought a rat and a snake and tossed them into his room. It was a non-venomous snake, but I feel sure that the poor old official did not know that at the time. The boxing squad is probably better remembered for the injustice done to Jeff Fenech. In the quarter-finals the judges gave the flyweight bout to Fenech over Redzep Redzepovski of Yuglosavia 3–2. Unbelievably, a jury reversed the decision and awarded the fight to the veteran Yugoslav 4–1. In the final Redzepovski was beaten by Steve McCrory (USA) and had the hide to complain, 'As long as an American is standing on his feet for three rounds it's hard to get a decision over him.' Fenech had the last laugh though. In disgust he immediately turned professional and went on to win world titles in three different weight divisions (and among the beaten challengers was LA gold medal winner McCrory).

IN 1988 AT the Seoul Games I was involved with the soccer team, the first time an Australian team had been in the Olympics since 1956. The team did quite well beating Yugoslavia and Nigeria, each by 1–0, and losing 3–0 to the highly favoured and subsequent runners-up Brazil in the preliminary rounds. The Socceroos then went down 3–0 in the quarter-finals to the Soviet Union, who went on to win gold. The Australians were eventually rated as fifth in the tournament.

The soccer venues were not only in Seoul, but spread all over South Korea in different centres. When the team was first in Seoul I used to wander down to the athletes' training oval where the monosyllabic Canadian sprint star, Ben Johnson, would be preparing for the sprints.

One look and there was no doubt that he was pumped up on steroids. It turned out that he was taking a steroid called stanozolol, which his doctor used to discontinue some time before an event to get it out of his system, thereby avoiding a positive drug test. Ben became disappointed with his form and decided, presumably without his coach or doctor realising, to go back on it again. On the day of the eagerly anticipated 100m race, the Australian soccer team was far away in the southern city of Pusan, but were able to watch the big event on television. Johnson won easily in world record time. The discovery of drugs in his system saw to it that he did not hold either his title or his record for very long, and had to leave Seoul in disgrace.

My other job, when we finally returned to Seoul from Pusan, was with the boxing — a job I was given because no one else wanted it. The boxing tournament turned out to be the greatest shambles you could ever imagine for the simple reason that many officials remarkably saw the bouts involving South Koreans very differently to the experts in the media — Koreans who were hammered mercilessly somehow ended up winning their bouts. The Koreans were definite they had been handed a very raw deal by the Americans four years before and seemed very determined to make up for it. And make up for it they did.

In the final of the light-middleweight division, the 19-year-old American Roy Jones Junior simply annihilated Park Si-hun, his (at-best) mediocre opponent who hardly struck a blow. Despite this Park was awarded the gold medal. Jones had suspected this would happen. Three days before the bout he had told journalists, 'I know how tough it is to get a decision against a South Korean, but it doesn't matter. If they cheat me, that's OK. I'll know if I really won it.' Indeed, Park had won each of his lead-up fights in disputed decisions, so much so that the media had laughingly been describing him as 'the unbeatable Park'.

Compubox, a computer company using software to tally clean punches that connected, registered 86 for Jones and 32 for Park. The headline on the story of the bout in the famous French sporting newspaper *L'Equipe* roughly translated as, 'So scandalous — to vomit'. Even the Korean fighter himself was embarrassed and told Jones, 'I lost the fight. I am sorry.' Ironically, Jones was later awarded the Val Barker Trophy that goes to the most outstanding boxer at each Olympics.

The incredible decision was never reversed and, as far as I know, Park never fought again. The universal outrage forced the International

Boxing Federation to radically change the scoring system, which is now decided by judges electronically registering clean blows. If a majority of the judges press their button simultaneously, a point is recorded and a screen in the arena lets everyone know. If there are any shenanigans the fans quickly voice their displeasure.

It wasn't only the boxers themselves who were affected at Seoul. Even worse was the treatment handed out by the Koreans to the New Zealand referee, Keith Walker, a really nice, sincere guy. Following a fairly rough bantamweight fight, Bulgarian Alexander Hristov, one of the favourites for the title, was given the points decision over the South Korean Byun Jong-il. After many warnings for head-butting, Byun failed to stop these tactics and Walker twice ordered a point to be deducted from his score. This ultimately cost him the bout. The Korean trainer, followed by other team officials, jumped into the ring and the angry Koreans rained blows down on the hapless New Zealander and tried to kick him. One of them pulled out a large lump of his hair. There were some security guards, but they began punching and kicking

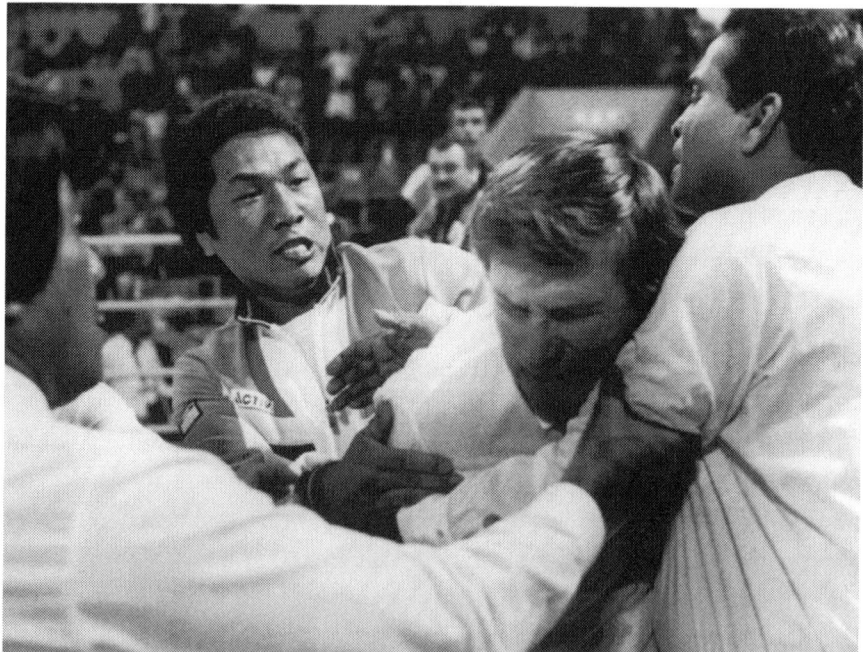

At the 1988 Seoul Olympics, referee Keith Walker was attacked by South Korean team members after their boxer, bantamweight Byun Jong-II, was beaten by Bulgarian boxer Alexander Hristov on a points decision. (AAP IMAGE/AFP)

Walker too. Walker had had enough; he left the stadium, checked out of his hotel, caught a taxi to the airport and flew back to New Zealand. The Korean boxer staged a silent sit-down strike in the middle of the ring, hunched up all alone, for 67 minutes.

Eventually, the Korean government officially apologised to the New Zealand government for all the misbehaving and the head of the Korean Olympics Committee resigned. It was the least he could do.

Lithgow fighter Grahame 'Spike' Cheney went close to winning Australia's first gold medal in the ring. He fought his way through to the final in the light-welterweight division after beating opponents from Paraguay, Ghana, the United States and Sweden (luckily he didn't come up against any South Koreans). Sadly, Cheney went down in the final to an experienced Soviet fighter Viatcheslav Yanovski and had to be content with a silver medal.

An interesting name among the boxers who fought at the Seoul Olympics was one that meant nothing at all to Australians at the time. It does now. Kostya Tszyu. In the lightweight division he was eliminated by the eventual gold medal winner, East German Andreas Zuelow. Two judges awarded the fight to Zuelow, two to Tszyu and the fifth, from Iraq, scored it a draw. Under the intriguing rules at that time a judge was not allowed to give a draw, so the Iraqi gave his vote to Zuelow. It was one of only 11 losses in 270 amateur bouts fought by Tszyu.

Debbie Flintoff-King produced one of the finest finishes in any Olympic athletics event coming from fourth place with two obstacles remaining to win the 400-metre hurdles and gold for Australia.

An added note on the women's hockey side achieving the ultimate at these games. They came up against South Korea in the final, played before a xenophobic local crowd of more than 26,000. The Koreans had been offered a pension of $US1000 per month for life if they won, a massive amount of money in that country. The Australians were unmoved, coming out 2–0 winners.

QUITE A FEW awards and honours have come my way over the years, but I do not think any of them could ever beat carrying the Olympic torch on its journey to the Sydney Olympics. The first Olympics were held in 776 BC in a remote area in the valley of Olympia. It was a sacred site for Greeks dedicated to the worship of the God of Gods, Zeus. The torch

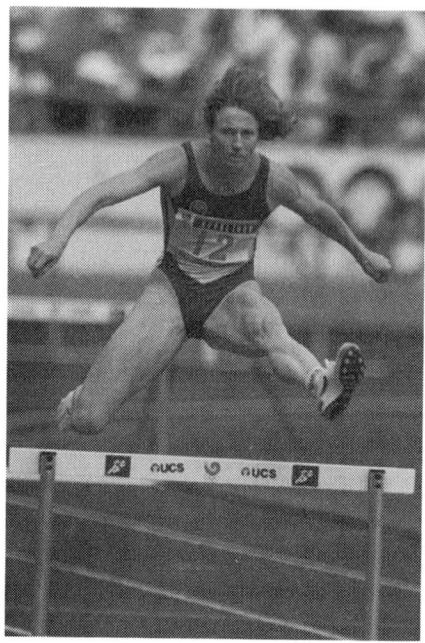
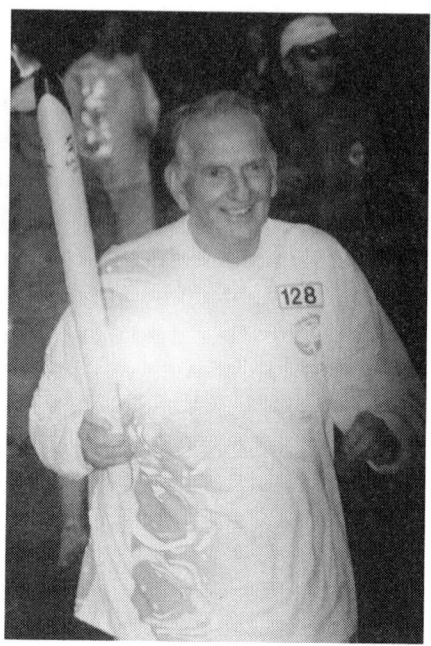

(LEFT) **Australian Debbie Flintoff-King hurdles to victory at the 1988 Seoul Olympics.** (AAP IMAGE/ SPORT THE LIBRARY) **Nothing can beat carrying the Olympic torch. I carried it at Cessnock, NSW, on its way to the 2000 Sydney Olympics.** (BRIAN CORRIGAN'S COLLECTION)

was first lit in those days to symbolise the death and rebirth of Greek heroes, but now, nearly 3000 years later, it represents an eternal light symbolising peace and great athletic performances.

The section I was to run in 2000 was on 29 August at Cessnock, north of Sydney, towards the end of the eighty-third day. I travelled there with some friends and family. The whole organisation of the torch carrying was military-like in its precision, even the cops went out of their way to be friendly. Carrying the torch might not sound particularly inspiring, but here, in my imagination at least, I had a feeling of being linked with the long history of past Olympics and with all the other lucky ones who had been carrying it. If you think I am going a bit over the top, let me tell you there were a lot of others out there who reported exactly the same feeling. It was such an honour to carry the torch.

The flame is extinguished at the end of each Olympics. Before the next Olympics a new flame is lit in an elaborate ceremony in Olympia, using a special mirror to focus the sun's rays. The idea of lighting the flame was revived in 1928, but the first torch relay was only initiated for the 1936 Berlin Olympics. You can easily imagine it being enthusiastically taken up by the Nazi regime.

In May 2000, the flame was lit in Olympia for the Sydney Games. From there the torch travelled to the Athens stadium where the first modern Olympics had been held in 1896, and from there around Greece for 10 days. It was then flown across the equator to Guam before being carried around New Zealand and 10 other Pacific nations.

An Australian design, the torch was a symbol of Sydney with the sails of the Opera House curving in the shape of a boomerang. It was coloured blue to represent the Pacific Ocean and was 72 centimetres long and weighed about 1 kilogram. It was designed to resist high winds, rain and being held upside down. It was seen in nearly all of Australia and played a big role in stimulating public interest in the Olympics and created incredible patriotic fervor in the huge, good-natured and well-behaved crowds that flocked into Sydney for each day of the Games.

All types of people were involved in carrying the torch. The young and the elderly — one man was 100 years old, bless him — some people were in wheelchairs, some were fit, some were fat. The torch was carried over mountains, across deserts, on horseback, on camels, by surfboat, and across the Great Barrier Reef by a scuba diver (an incredible technical feat as the torch was underwater for 3 minutes).

On 8 June it arrived at Uluru in the middle of the red heart of Australia, where the Governor-General, Sir William Deane, and the traditional Aboriginal owners greeted their 'firestick'. In the first leg of the relay the torch was carried, among others, by tennis champion, Evonne Goolagong-Cawley and athlete Nova Peris, our first indigenous gold medal winner (in the Atlanta hockey side) who, with her nine-year-old daughter, ran barefoot as a mark of respect for the sacred site, Uluru. Then it was flown to the Alice where, considering the size of the town, an amazing 15,000 people greeted it.

The torch later zigzagged across Australia for 27,000 kilometres, the longest single distance the flame had ever travelled — 100 days, with 8500 carriers at an average of 100 people a day, with 2500 schoolchildren as escort runners. All previous Australian Olympians, sponsors and Games staff along with certain privileged people were invited to apply to run with the torch, including one sportsman who was in jail for drug running. When he received his invitation he said that he would jump at the opportunity to run. The authorities, possibly misunderstanding him, wouldn't let him out for the day.

Great care was taken to avoid the prank played in Sydney in 1956 when some 400,000 people lined the Olympic torch route from Hornsby. The 'torch' arrived at Sydney Town Hall some 11 minutes early and was greeted by the then Lord Mayor of Sydney, Pat Hills, who was well into his welcoming speech before it was realised it was a hoax. Everybody thought it was all highly amusing, save the Lord Mayor. A university student had perpetrated the prank using a jam tin on a stick.

On the day I was to carry the torch, the runners were all assembled in Cessnock and then driven by bus to the various set-down points along the route to wait for the first sight of the oncoming runner. A convoy of about 50 vehicles, including police escorts, security and backups, followed behind. Schoolchildren escorts, about a dozen of them, all dressed in their blue uniforms, jogged merrily along beside this cavalcade for kilometres, seemingly inexhaustible.

I had two problems with the run. The first was the run was uphill; the second that it all seemed a blur and was over so quickly. I wished it could have lasted so much longer. The greatest thrill, and the one I will never forget, was when the bus picked us up after the run and drove us back to Cessnock, where we were greeted not only by family and friends, but hordes of schoolchildren all wanting their photo taken with the torch. Torch-bearers were given a replica of the real one, when I said they could take mine to get their photo taken, their eyes shone like sparklers. They lined up with every available relative, a never-to-be-forgotten moment. That night ended with a gigantic barbecue at the local park organised by the locals and attended by more people than the usual population of Cessnock itself.

For the torch to travel all around Australia, without a hitch, was a huge accomplishment and a tribute to all those who organised it. I'm quite certain every single person who carried the torch also has in his or her home a memento of that highly successful and meaningful day. I absolutely loved the whole experience.

'Jim Bayutti was a flamboyant, larger-than-life, love him or hate him (and no in-between) kind of guy ... one of the greatest characters I have ever met.'

18. IF HE'S FROM APIA, PICK HIM

MY WORK AT Arsenal — from 1961 to 1963 — eventually attracted the attention of soccer authorities back in Australia. In 1967, a couple of years after my eventual return home to Sydney, I had a visit from Aussie soccer chief Jim (Giacomo) Bayutti. He was headhunting, and I was in his sights.

At that stage soccer in Australia boasted the highest profile of its 80-year history, but the popularity had come at a cost. There had been a breakaway from the ruling body, the Australian Soccer Association, in 1957 and the Australian Soccer Federation was formed. The new clubs looked to Europe for talent but could not afford the transfer fees being asked for. Some clubs illegally poached stars such as the trio from the FK Austria club in Vienna — Karl Jaros, Leo Baumgartner and Walter Tamandl. As a result of this, the world's governing body Fédération Internationale de Football Association (FIFA) decided, in 1959, to suspend Australia from international competition. A peace agreement was eventually negotiated in 1963 with the Australian Soccer Federation paying FIFA £25,000 (AUD$50,000) as compensation for the unpaid transfer fees.

Now, back in the international fold, Australia had ambitions of reaching the World Cup finals. And Jim Bayutti was at the forefront of the drive. He was the man behind the formation of one of Australia's most famous soccer and social clubs APIA (Associazione Polisportiva Italo-Australiana, or Italian-Australian All Sports Association), a decade earlier. With Sir Stanley Rous, then president of FIFA and Sid Guppy, the chairman of the New Zealand Football Association, Bayutti laid the foundations for the formation of the Oceania Football Confederation in 1966, through which Australia hoped to qualify for the World Cup finals.

Bayutti was a flamboyant, larger-than-life, love him or hate him (and no in-between) kind of guy. He was definitely one of the greatest characters I have ever met. As President of the Australian Soccer Federation he was at the centre of intense internal wrangling. His bitter battles with his successor, Sir Arthur George, were regularly splashed across the sporting pages of the nation's newspapers and never helped the cause of soccer.

Like thousands of other Italians, Jim had emigrated in the 1950s to work on the giant Snowy Mountains Scheme. He quickly made a name for himself among his fellow migrant workers on the Snowy and set up his own construction firm. Among the company's projects was work building the Sydney Opera House. It was not long before Bayutti was a millionaire. He had several passions in life — his family, APIA and soccer.

At the time he strode into my life I was tied up with the Australian Rugby League. I had become quite disenchanted because, friendly as the League chiefs were, their ideas were firmly rooted in the past with no real desire to see any change. I had come back from England with lots of ideas about treating injuries, improving training methods and even methods of promoting the game. Bill Buckley, the League president, would listen to me patiently, say he agreed with everything, but nothing ever changed because that was not the way it had been done for the last 40 years or so. The League hierarchy seemed to be top-heavy with former front-row forwards. There was a running joke that unless you had put your head into at least 2000 scrums you wouldn't be considered for any senior position with the Rugby League.

If I may say so, it is amazing to see how many of my ideas about training, weight training for one, have since been adopted by Rugby League coaches.

I told Jim about my experiences. His reply was that I was exactly the person he was looking for and asked was there anything I could think of to help soccer? In those days, there was a definite lack of fitness in all the football clubs and I said that the Australian soccer team should have a fitness program. The players also needed to be regularly tested for fitness to assess their progress.

Bayutti issued an edict on the spot. I would arrange to do the assessments with coach Joe Vlasits and that future representative teams would be selected only on the basis of those fitness tests. That was exactly what I wanted to hear, so I readily agreed to become the Soccer Federation's doctor.

Jim said he was going on a visit to Italy for a month, returning in time for one of New South Wales' matches against Manchester United, who were touring Australia fresh from winning England's League Championship, at the Sydney Showground.

The testing required a great deal of work. We checked every candidate for the squad, grading the players in each playing position in order of their degree of fitness. Joe Vlasits was particularly happy because all the old guard of players, whom he intended to sack anyway, came out far and away the worst in the fitness tests.

We met with Bayutti after he returned from his trip, and were sitting up the back of the stand one night while the squad was training. The meeting lasted about one minute. Jim handed us a sheet of paper and noted, 'I've picked the team for the weekend, here it is.'

Joe and I looked at each other in disbelief. We were aghast. So much for picking teams on the basis of fitness, or that we would be joint selectors with him. Vlasits read out the team sheet. It listed most of the players he was trying to drop. As you might imagine, they were mainly APIA players.

With considerable irony, Joe added, 'You haven't picked a goalkeeper.'

Bayutti didn't even blink, 'Oh, haven't I? What's the name of the APIA goalie, Joe?'

Joe told him, and Bayutti added it to the list. With the team finalised, Jim made some comment about being a busy man, got to his feet and left.

Joe and I sat looking at each other and I suggested the only thing to do was to resign immediately. He said it would be better for us to hang in there. Maybe things would improve with time.

Jim Bayutti was the type of man I couldn't help but like. Joe felt the same way, so we made it up with him while demanding there was to be no repeat of such high-handed behaviour.

'Most definitely!' Jim assured us.

We did not have too much time to test him out, for he did not last much longer. He lost his boardroom battle with Sir Arthur and was deposed. Bayutti died, painfully, of throat cancer not long afterwards, very much mourned by a host of friends.

For the record: Manchester United won the match 3–1 (and a second one a couple of days later 3–0). During the game, in which John Warren was captain for the first time and some 30,000 exuberant fans packed the arena, Denis Law, United's Scottish international and European Footballer of the Year in 1964, thought he was too important to be receiving the close marking he was getting from our Ron Giles. So he head-butted Giles, fracturing his cheekbone. Charming!

Oh, yes ... and I always remember that the APIA goalie's name had definitely not been on our list.

LOVABLE UNCLE JOE

Joe Vlasits was known to all and sundry as 'Uncle Joe' because that's what he was like, everyone's favourite uncle. He was born in Hungary and played professional football there. After his playing career finished he became the national youth coach and a selector for the national senior side.

Uncle Joe migrated to Sydney in 1949 with his wife Chibby. His impeccable credentials ensured he was snapped up as coach of the Prague club. Vlasits then switched to Canterbury where he introduced an incredibly successful youth policy putting together a team that was known affectionately as the 'Canterbury Babes'. Several of the Vlasits-groomed youngsters became household names in soccer, including John Warren and John Watkiss. The 'Babes' did extraordinarily well winning the Federation Championship in 1958 and 1960 and the Ampol Cup in 1958. Joe had stints at various other clubs before taking on the national coaching job.

Uncle Joe was instrumental in forming the Soccer Coaches Federation. I had first met him in 1965 not long after I came back from the United Kingdom. He was impressed with my ideas and asked me to give lectures to the coaching fraternity.

The former Yugal star Tiko Jelisavcic had captained the players in Australia's first attempt at the World Cup, losing two matches in 1965

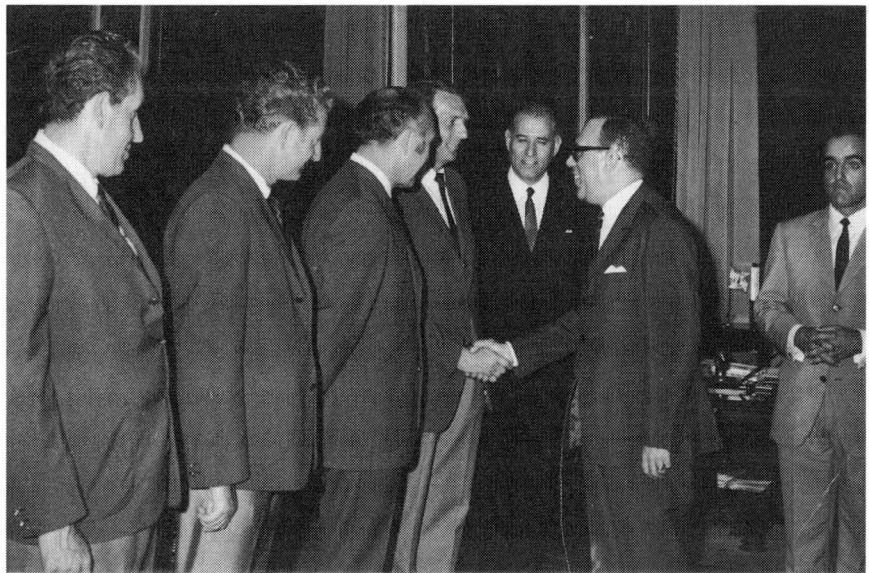

Members of the Australian support staff meet the Portuguese Governor in Mozambique, 1969. Coach Joe Vlasits is on the left, Tom Patrick (Qantas), Les Bordacs (manager), and I am shaking his hand. (BRIAN CORRIGAN'S COLLECTION)

against North Korea (6–1 and 3–1). As neither side had diplomatic recognition of the other, the 'home and away' matches were both played in the Cambodian capital of Phnom Penh (the real winner was the Cambodian government, which slapped a 29.5 per cent tax on the gate takings). Jelisavcic was shown the door when he failed to get the Aussies through to the finals. His successor, Joe Venglos, had only a brief stint before leaving Australia when he could not get official recognition of his academic qualifications.

Uncle Joe, an ideal man for the job, took over after Venglos' departure in 1967 and continued his youth policy with his international selections. In his first foray overseas most of the players were around 20 years of age and the two oldest were just 26. They were to form the basis of our World Cup teams in the 1970s. His players loved him even though he was an 'olde worlde' type of guy and spoke fractured English with many unique and quite strange expressions. Some people may have laughed behind his back at the way he spoke. I certainly never did. Indeed, I have fond memories of the way Uncle Joe would regularly turn to me and ask, 'Vot you tink, Brian?'

A great guy!

'There were people looking under our bus with mirrors to check if any mines had been planted.'

19. THE KY TO VICTORY

IT'S NOW UNIVERSALLY accepted that the Vietnam War was one of the great political mistakes of history. Ho Chi Minh, a nom de guerre translated as 'he who enlightens', had led the resistance to the Japanese occupation during World War II. He claimed the Americans had promised his people self-government in return for their help in beating the Japanese. Instead the French had claimed their colony back after the War.

Uncle Ho, as he was affectionately named by his followers, then turned his efforts against the French who were forced to quit the country after a massive defeat at the hands of the Viet Minh in the Battle of Dien Bien Phu in 1954. The ensuing peace treaty reached in negotiations with French Prime Minister Pierre Mendes-France divided the country into North Vietnam and South Vietnam along the 17th parallel. It was an arrangement that was never going to succeed.

In 1960, the Viet Cong (VC), the military arm of the National Liberation Front in the North, crossed the 17th parallel and infiltrated South Vietnam. In 1962 US President John F Kennedy supplied a few thousand military advisors to stiffen the resolve of South Vietnam's army. President Lyndon Johnson increased this to 75,000 American ground troops in 1965 and then to 500,000 by 1968. The ensuing political turmoil resulted in the loss of his Presidency that year.

The Australian Prime Minister, Sir Robert Menzies, had also agreed to send 30 military advisors in 1962, introduced conscription in 1964 and committed troops to fight the following year. In 1966, his successor

Harold Holt trebled the number and the first conscripts went off to fight amid violent protests by anti-Vietnam War demonstrators.

AMID THIS UPHEAVAL, you might well ask what on earth we were doing taking a young soccer team to war-ravaged Saigon, the capital of South Vietnam, in November 1967? It seemed crazy, risking the lives of these young Australian sportsmen, but Australia's Department of Foreign Affairs decided that it would be a good idea for our team to compete in the Friendship Tournament to be held between various friendly South-East Asian and Pacific countries: New Zealand, Thailand, Malaya, Singapore, South Korea, Hong Kong, and Australia as well as South Vietnam. The tournament would coincide with South Vietnam's National Day. Some of us thought it was like waving a red rag at the Viet Cong.

We took this young team under our coach, Joe Vlasits. We also had a physiotherapist, two journalists, one referee and my great friend, Tom Patrick, who worked for Qantas and was there as its travel consultant. This team would end up forming the nucleus of the team that would play for a spot in the World Cup two years later. There were some of the

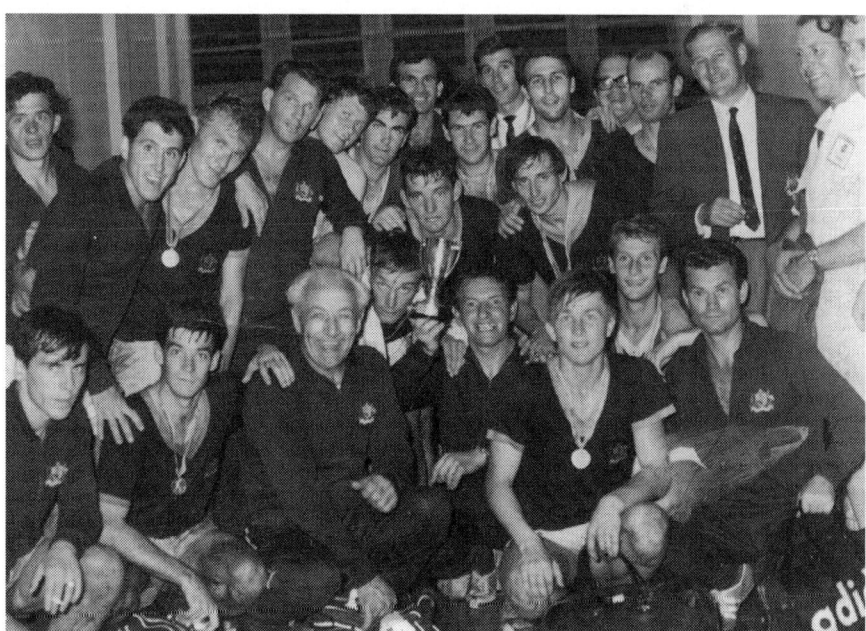

The Australian soccer team after winning the final, November 1967.
(BRIAN CORRIGAN'S COLLECTION)

greats of Australia's soccer history, including Manfred Schaefer, Atti Abonyi, John Warren, Ray Baartz and Ray Richards.

What an extraordinary feeling it was to fly into Saigon's Tan Son Nhut Airport, packed with warplanes almost wing tip to wing tip, with the sound of distant (and sometimes not so distant) guns and mortars.

Nothing could have prepared us for our hotel, which for some strange reason had been called the Golden Building. Golden it most certainly was not! As we walked through the door I thought, 'What a funny thing to do, bringing us in through such a filthy basement.' It turned out to be the main reception area. Our fullback, Stan Ackerley, walked into his room to switch on the light and was thrown right across the room. The light switch had bare wires poking out from it. Abonyi shared his room with a giant lizard.

It had been a long flight from Sydney, so the first thing for a tired and hungry team was to get lunch. On a large plate was a small slice of something I presumed to be greasy Spam. Nothing else.

'No,' snarled the surly hotel owner. 'That is all you can get because you are issued with food coupons and there are no more left for this meal.'

It quickly became apparent that the proprietor had already taken his cut. If we wanted any more we were going to have to come to some arrangement with him. There was another problem, this time with fluids. The players were under strict instructions — no ice and no drink that wasn't bottled, but most of the local soft drink bottles had a thick, black rim of grease around the top. Yuk! We did get some better soft drink bottles by exchanging some of the food coupons. I can report that as team doctor I was able to survive on beer.

The New Zealand team manager was Jack Cowie. As a young man he had been one of their Test cricket team's finest medium-paced bowlers, but it seemed to us he was a disaster as a manager. His first directive was that there was no need to avoid ice. After a few days, the illnesses started and the Kiwis had to go looking for a doctor. For one game they had only ten fit players and eventually one player was so ill that he was left in a Vietnamese hospital while the rest returned home. We never had any stomach problems on the entire tour.

The day after we arrived, we were given a briefing by staff from the Australian Embassy.

'Be very careful of people on bikes, especially if they have women on the back, as they may think you are an American and shoot you, and be very careful, as people plant a number of nasty anti-personnel mines around the place. All playing fields will be combed for mines before you play.'

When we got outside the embassy it seemed all of Saigon was riding around on bikes with women on the back and there were people looking under our bus with mirrors to check if any mines had been planted. It was not particularly reassuring. Most of the team had been quite blasé about being in a war zone. Now they had suddenly gone quiet.

We had security on every floor of our building, and every morning our chief security man would come in and park his guns in the corner. His name was Hung, so the team nicknamed him 'Well'. When he arrived they always greeted him with: 'Well, Hung.' He was never sure why they would dissolve into laughter, so he used to laugh along with them.

A GREAT DEAL is heard these days, especially in Rugby League, about the need for bonding, which seems to be little more than an excuse to get together and drink a lot of grog. The bonding of the Australian soccer team in those Spartan conditions in Saigon left a legacy of team spirit, the will to win and a pride that has lasted right up to this day, but this didn't just happen. It was carefully nurtured by coach Joe Vlasits, who went out of his way to make everyone there feel that they were each an important cog in the team.

The Golden Building was so dreadful that we decided to leave the owner to gloat over his few measly coupons and find another place to eat. We were saved by the Australian Army. Tom Patrick found someone he knew who readily organised for us to eat with them at the Army's 'Canberra Club' where facilities were excellent and there were also areas for the boys to relax playing games such as table tennis.

The 'Canberra Club' had sandbag bunkers outside the building, guarded by two soldiers with rifles, whose brief was to ensure that the traffic kept flowing in the street we were in. They did not want the Viet Cong to be able to pause outside to throw a bomb. If the traffic slowed, they would shoot once in the air. Apparently, if the traffic didn't improve in a hurry, the soldiers were allowed to shoot the offenders on the spot. The air around our haven of relaxation would always be punctuated by the sound of guns going off just behind our ears.

Later, some of us were invited to the very upmarket American Officers' Club, but I didn't enjoy that much at all. The sight of huge steaks and lobsters, all washed down with a selection of excellent wines, together with mounds of ice-cream, did not sit too well while the television sets were bragging about the enemy body count for the day and the poverty and hardships all around us. One of my overriding impressions was just how much the Americans spoke about the Vietnamese in derogatory terms. Most of them seemed to hate or at least look down on the local population.

MATCHES IN THE Friendship Tournament at the Cong Hoa Stadium were usually played in mud that came up to our ankles. The huge crowds were always against us, except for when we played South Korea, whose excessively brutal, ruthless troops were loathed more than other foreign soldiers there … and that is saying something!

We beat New Zealand 5–3 with Abonyi netting three goals and Warren and Baartz one apiece. Our next opponent was the host nation, South Vietnam. It is almost impossible, even today, to convey what the atmosphere and the noise were like. Soldiers with fixed bayonets were everywhere, barbed wire, army snipers and outside the stadium, army personnel carriers. There was a near riot after Warren had scored a sensational goal to give us a 1–0 lead just before half-time. The use of tear gas was even discussed. The Prime Minister, Air Vice-Marshal Nguyen Cao Ky was at the game and during the disturbance those of us down on the bench were ordered to move up into the stand and sit just behind Ky. I thought it would be as a good a time as ever, amid all this pandemonium, for someone to assassinate him, then quickly realised if they were aiming at him they would just as likely shoot me instead. During the half-time break Ky went down to South Vietnam's dressing-room and offered them a small fortune to win, but this ended up having the opposite effect. Our team heard about Ky's offer and were doubly determined to hold onto their lead, which they did.

The Vietnamese were incurable gamblers. The main reason for the crowd disturbance was almost certainly not their patriotic fervour, but the money they had gambled on the home team which looked like losing.

The manner in which our team handled the difficult conditions was most impressive. They did not appear to have a care in the world. At one stage I had to go onto the field to treat an injury, and some of the players were singing to themselves the team song. The words were about Australians being 'Cheap Charlies' (meaning they wouldn't buy the bar girls of Saigon a drink of the brown-coloured water they were selling and claiming to be whisky).

Once the game was over, we were told to wait in the dressing shed for a short time while the army and police dispersed the crowd. We were more than happy to obey!

The Australians went on to beat Singapore 5–1 with another hat-trick to Abonyi and with Baartz and Warren each scoring a goal. In the semi-finals we overcame Malaysia 1–0 thanks to a Baartz goal while South Korea beat the home side 3–0. In the final attended by both Ky and President Nguyen Van Thieu, we accounted for South Korea 3–2 with Billy Vojtek, Abonyi and Warren scoring the goals.

On the way home we played a few more games, beating Indonesia 2–0 and 3–1 in Jakarta, then another three wins, beating Singapore 6–1 in Singapore and Malaysia 4–0 in Kuala Lumpur. Atti Abonyi ended up with eleven goals in his eight matches.

SELECTION BUNGLE AT VUNG TAU

A day after our last game in Saigon, we were due to fly to Vung Tau, a coastal town, that Australian soldiers used for R & R — rest and recreation. We intended to have a relaxing day with the troops, some sun, sand and swimming. And, of course, a barbecue.

I wondered aloud if 'Charlie' (the American and Australian army slang for the Viet Cong) ever disrupted these peaceful proceedings. The Aussie soldiers assured me it never happened, because the Viet Cong also used Vung Tau for the same recreational purposes.

The team was also going to play a game of soccer against an Australian Army selection, which would give everybody in our squad of 18 a bit of a run. A few minutes before the end, the score was 10–0 our way. I saw there might be a chance for me to get on the field for a few minutes, so I could boast to incredulous friends that I had once played soccer for Australia. My friend Uncle Joe said that he could never allow the standard to sink that low. So I missed out.

To reach Vung Tau we had to get up early to catch a plane from Tan Son

Nhut Airport. Celebrating our victory of the night before, we stayed up late and had a few beers, then some more, and after that a few more. It got so late we decided to stay up all night. We were a particularly seedy group at the airport. We became distinctly seedier when we saw our transport, a Caribou airplane. We met the two pilots; they seemed very friendly, normal sort of guys, but, oh, so very young.

We climbed in through the open back of the aircraft, sat against the wall of the plane and strapped ourselves in. The take off seemed a bit rough, although that may only have been our imagination, but it definitely became rough as we stared out of the back of the plane at the rapidly receding ground while the plane continued to toss violently from side to side. We were sick enough before we got into the air, but to be staring out the open back of a plane seemingly being piloted by a couple of gung-ho madmen was too much. Everyone looked paler than the white tuxedo Frank Sinatra used to wear.

It got worse. When we arrived, one of the fresh-faced pilots decided to buzz the beach. He flew so low I swear that the soldiers bathing in the ocean were ducking their heads. We thought that was funny and so apparently did the pilot, who decided we might like to see it again, so he circled and repeated the procedure.

Great treatment for a hangover!

'Once he was in a helicopter and the Viet Cong were shooting through the floor. I began to understand his paranoia.'

20. JACK THE QUACK

THE VIETNAM WAR always seemed to be so horribly pointless. Unwinnable, no matter how many American troops were thrown in, it exacted a terrible price not only for those who died on all sides (and their families) but afterwards as well when so many fell victim to psychological trauma. Such a fate befell Dr Jack Blomley.

Jack, from Tumbarumba in southern New South Wales, was one of my good mates at St Joseph's boarding school in Sydney, a happy-go-lucky individual with never a care or worry in the world. He took these attributes on to the sporting field, where he was a very fine athlete excelling at rugby union and cricket. In the rugby first XV team he played under the famous Brother Henry whose most recent teams included future Test players in Arthur Tonkin, Brian Piper and Paul Johnson. Brother Henry told us that Jack was the most natural five-eighth he ever had. Jack Blomley was also a good cricketer, playing in the first XI and GPS firsts. I actually thought he was a better cricketer, especially as a fine swing bowler, than a football player, but he rarely put his mind to it. I played a game with him once at university. The first five balls he faced he hit for four. He snicked the next. He also excelled in many other sports.

Blomley studied medicine after leaving school, so I saw a fair bit of him, as we were in the same year at Sydney University. While there he played seven Tests as centre for Australia at rugby union (alongside the great Trevor Allan against the New Zealand Maoris and the All Blacks in 1949 and, after Allan switched to rugby league, with Alan Walker against the 1950 British Lions). He would have made the 1947–48 tour of Britain but suffered a severe ankle injury. We used to practise with him walking straight without a limp up and down the corridor in the Medical School. He said that the medical examination for the tour was hopeless and if he could walk in without a limp he would pass it. It was not to be. He kept playing but unfortunately in the end it did cut his career short.

Our last meeting at university says a lot about Jack. That day we were both sitting up the back of one of the classes. This class was the only one in the medical course where you had to sign an attendance book. Every student had to attend at least 25 lectures before being allowed to sit for the exams. As fate would have it, on this very last day of term, both Jack and I had attended 24 times. Jack hadn't reached the magic figure because he had been away playing rugby union for Australia in the Shaky Isles (New Zealand) and in my case … well, I had been doing other things. Jack was telling me about the great football he had played across the ditch. The lecturer was getting a bit irate about our talking, not that I had any chance to shut Jack up. He told me that after one Test he had come off the field black and blue. Did I know why? No, I didn't know why.

'Well,' said Jack, earnestly. 'I not only had to tackle my man but I had to tackle [winger] Johnny Solomon's man too.'

I couldn't help myself and burst out laughing.

'You, out!' roared the voice from the front. The lecturer was pointing at me.

I was devastated. I had just blown my last chance to sit for the exams. But I was saved … by Jack. He went up to the lecturer to say he had picked the wrong man, that it really was him. Jack charmed him with stories about what a great football player he was. The result? We both got to sign the book and I did not have to face the prospect of having to explain what happened when I got home.

You need friends like that in life.

I lost contact with Jack Blomley after we graduated. He first went to work with the flying doctor in Western Australia for a year or more before settling in Stockton, a working-class suburb in Newcastle. He married Maureen, had five children and ran a large general practice. He also joined the Civilian Military Force (CMF) as a doctor. When the

Vietnam War started he volunteered to go, even though he could easily have got an exemption because of his large family. Jack said he felt it was his duty since he was a member of the CMF.

Soon after we arrived in Saigon, I had to arrange for an X-ray on John Watkiss's leg. The only place we could get one was at the huge American hospital not far away from our hotel. Just as John and I were going through the hospital gates, whom did we meet but Jack! I must say I was very glad to see, not only someone I knew and remembered so fondly, someone who could also help us find our way around.

His initial, urgent greeting was, 'Get down you bloody fool, don't you realise they could zap you?'

'Who will?' I said, looking about.

'They have snipers on the roofs and they can zap you.'

I didn't take it any further even though I wanted to ask who exactly 'they' were (I did have a pretty good idea). Jack quickly took me by the arm and rushed us inside the hospital.

He asked, 'How are you going to get back to your hotel?'

'The same way we got here. In the bus.'

'You can't take a bus, they could zap you on the way. I've got my car and driver here. I'll drive you back.'

At this stage my old friend still had not even said hello to either of us. After we came back from the X-ray department, I was thankful Jack was waiting. Off we drove in his jeep with Jack anxiously scanning the rooftops, hardly saying a word.

We were approaching a huge five-way intersection, with massive transport trucks coming and going on all sides, when Jack said to his Vietnamese driver, 'Don't stop.'

'But I might have to stop,' came the reply.

Now I have to tell you that the Vietnamese police (or 'White Mice' as they were called because of their distinctive white jackets) were a law unto themselves. They would blow their whistle, shoot once in the air and, because of Viet Cong infiltrators, if you didn't immediately obey them then they could shoot you. No questions asked.

We were getting close to the intersection when the White Mouse on point duty turned towards us and put his hand up to stop.

'I have to stop,' wailed the driver in a panic-stricken voice, while Jack's two passengers in the back silently nodded in agreement. Jack pulled out his service revolver, held it at the head of the driver, who was now sweating profusely, and roared, 'Keep driving or I will shoot you.'

It was so bizarre that my first thought was that Jack was doing it for a joke or to scare us. The White Mouse was blowing his whistle and starting to reach for his gun. We had driven into the intersection with the huge transport trucks, three-abreast, bearing down on us from the right, at what seemed an alarming rate. The driver drove faster, the gun still at his head. I looked at Johnny Watkiss. He was a whiter shade of pale, as the Procul Harum hit song went. I'm sure I looked worse, John later told me he thought I had turned green. Two trucks whizzed a fraction past the back of us. The third truck, which also would not have stopped for us, passed within an inch of our back tyre. There was so much noise and confusion, I did not have time to wonder if the White Mouse was shooting of not.

We eventually arrived back at the Golden Building, with Johnny, the driver and me still shaking uncontrollably. Jack, on the other hand, seemed unconcerned about our experience.

Next day, Jack rang me up (and with not a single word about what had happened the day before) to invite me to visit him at his army clinic.

'OK, thanks, I'd love to,' I said. 'But if you don't mind I'll take a taxi.' He was fairly busy when I got there and in his own environment very much calmer, more like the old Jack I'd known in the past. Nobody had ever looked more unmilitary-like. The troops there called him Jack the Quack, but it was a term of endearment for they obviously thought the world of him. Jack loved them and his nickname in return. Some of the soldiers told me (he never mentioned it) he had been in an ambush twice and was more than fortunate to be alive. Once he was in a helicopter and the Viet Cong were shooting through the floor. I began to understand his paranoia.

Before each of our five games in Saigon I would invite Jack to come and watch us play. Every time he'd ask if the match in question was going to be played at night and when I said yes, he always came up with an excuse why he couldn't make it. Eventually it dawned on me that he was afraid of being out at night. When we reached the final against South Korea, I rang him and said I had a good idea — to save him travelling at night on his own, he could drive to our hotel around lunchtime, then come with us in the team bus and return to the hotel to stay with us for the night. Jack thought this was a great idea. He also said he would ask some of his army mates to come to the ground to be a cheer squad. I thought that was a good idea too, for supporters were very thin on the ground. Some other Australian soldiers turned up and another war almost erupted when they were refused admission. Finally after negotiations with the men on the gate we managed to squeeze them into one corner.

Jack duly turned up to our hotel when it was still daylight, but was obviously still anxious. He talked a lot, especially a lot about himself, and did not get on at all with our players, who wanted to know: 'Where did you get him from?'

'Give him a chance,' I told them. 'I'm sure he'll settle down.'

After we won the final, he came back with us on the team bus. We had dinner and decided to have a few beers. After a few drinks, a huge change came over Jack. He was his old self and was a huge success with the players, the life and soul of the party. They were even laughing at his stories and asking for more.

After some time, I noticed he was nowhere to be seen. I went searching around the building, but to no avail. There was no light in my room but I went in after I heard a bit of a noise. There was Jack, in the dark, curled up in a corner, crying his eyes out.

'Jack, mate, what's the matter?'

The answer from my boyhood hero really broke me up.

'Mate, I did not think that I could ever again be with a group of guys, just sitting around, having a few beers, having a normal conversation, cracking some jokes and bullshitting with them. I am so terribly grateful for what you have done for me tonight.'

It was my turn to cry.

He went on to explain that he could never sleep properly and felt certain the Viet Cong were trying to kill him. He always kept a gun under his pillow or by his side. Even when his wife had come to visit him when he was on R & R in Singapore, he had slept on the floor with the gun beside him.

When his tour of duty was over, Dr Jack Blomley returned home to Stockton. He still couldn't sleep, and died soon after from a coronary. All too young at just 46. A victim of the apocalyptic horror that was Vietnam.

THE DESERTER

While I was in Vietnam one of the Australian journalists in Saigon had a party in his flat one night and invited me along. It was a large flat on the main street, Tu Do, a wide, charming boulevard built by the French. There was plenty of food and drink, very nice music and quite a few men turned up. I say men, for, as you might imagine, there were few Western women anywhere in Saigon.

After a time, there was a loud banging on the door, and in barged a posse of White Mice.

'We are searching for an American deserter,' their leader shouted. Well, our host was most irate at this intrusion and told them in no uncertain terms that there was no way in the world anyone at the party would be harbouring an American deserter. He went on to warn that he was a very influential man and they had no right to be there. None of his posturing seemed to worry the White Mice at all. After a quick check on us they left, albeit grudgingly.

They had just gone out the front door of the building when one guest, who was more than a little intoxicated, leant over the balcony and poured a can of beer over them. Next thing, the door was again flung open and the White Mice stormed in with their guns drawn and fired a couple of shots into the lounge room ceiling. I kept as low a profile as humanly possible as, still brandishing their guns, the grim-faced White Mice randomly grabbed a couple of people and, screaming in Vietnamese, dragged them off to the local lock-up (although they weren't kept there very long, possibly because the police were still searching for the American deserter).

Just as things were beginning to settle down, an American voice suddenly said, 'That was the most stupid damn thing I have ever seen.'

'Where did you come from?' everyone said in unison.

'I've been hiding in the cupboard. Do you know, I could have been shot if they found me?'

He could have been shot? What about the rest of us?

The host was so furious that he could have shot the American himself. Instead he looked at the Yank, shrugged his shoulders and said, 'It's too late to worry about it now. You had better come and have a beer.'

'I am a lover and a poet, not a hero.'

21. THE RELUCTANT HERO

BRIAN (DEWEY) DEWHURST was a Sydney friend who worked for the United Press International (UPI) news agency, mainly as a tennis writer. He was a master of his craft. When I first met him, the stories told about the practical jokes he played, especially on his best friends, were legendary.

He was told he had to go to Vietnam as a war correspondent, which was a bitter blow for a sports writer. He thought he would most certainly die there. Before he left Sydney he gathered all his mates for a wake at which gave a farewell speech. The oration finished with the words: 'I don't know why I have to go, I am a lover and a poet, not a hero.'

While I was in Saigon we met up and Dewey told me about his arrival in Vietnam. On his first night he went out to dinner and, as usual, had drunk more than his share of the singing syrup. He had been warned that there was a strictly enforced curfew, that Australian soldiers guarded the place where he was staying and there was a password he would have to remember to get back in.

'No problem,' he told the officer who briefed him.

The officer reinforced the warning. Trip wires surrounded the place and if they were disturbed, flares would go off, there would be one shot in the air and he would have to sing out the password or else he would be shot.

'No problem,' Dewey said again, writing the password down on a piece of paper and shoving it one of his pockets.

When he did come back from his night out, and I know you can see this coming, Dewey stumbled over the trip wire and fell down, face first in the Saigon mud. Flares went up, one shot was fired and a voice shouted, 'Tell us the password.'

Of course, Dewey had forgotten the password and worse still he could not remember which pocket housed the piece of paper on which he had written it.

'Don't shoot me, I'm an Aussie and I've forgotten it.'

'Well, say something in Australian.'

'Johnny Raper,' Dewey shouted back, quoting the name of the legendary rugby league player.

'OK, mate. Come on in.'

When he told me the story I suggested he might be pulling my leg. A look of hurt spread across his face.

'Well, what would have happened to you if the soldier had come from Victoria?' I went on.

'That's easy. I'd have called out Ron Barassi!'

HE HAD ANOTHER story about an unusual nocturnal conversation.

The wife of a friend, who was also a renowned sports writer, suspected, and with very good cause, that the reason he was getting home so late at night was that he was fooling around where he should never have been fooling around. The sports writer's wife became tired of being home on her own and decided to do something about it by having a very late night out herself.

As luck would have it, her errant spouse got home quite early that particular evening and finding no wife, went to bed and fell sleep. He was woken up in the early hours, sat up in bed, and still half asleep thought he should make some sort of protest.

'Good heavens, Barbara [name changed], what's the score?'

'It's about one–all at this stage. One–all!'

DEWHURST LOVED THE English language, or should I say the Australian language. And not just because he earned his living by using it. He was particularly fond of rhyming slang, that wonderful Australian version of the expressions used by Cockneys. Rhyming slang probably arrived with those Cockneys unfortunate enough to be guests of His Majesty on the First Fleet and has changed subtly over ensuing generations. Whistle and Flute (suit) became Bag of Fruit. Butchers Hook (look) was changed to Captain Cook. And in the 1940s and 1950s several well-known Australian figures managed to get their names into rhyming slang, although they probably would have preferred not to. The Cockneys would refer to someone being Brahms and Listz (under the influence of alcohol). The Aussies, more of that in a moment. To go to the toilet, Aussies might well suggest they were going for a Johnny Bliss (named after a famed Sydney beach sprinter and footballer).

And so it was with Dewhurst. Only he would, at times, become quite obscure. He'd ask for a whisky with a dash of LKS. What was this LKS? The LKS Mackinnon Stakes (run on the Saturday before the Melbourne Cup), in distance it was a mile and a quarter, which rhymes with water. Hence a whisky with a dash of water.

Dewey was at Wimbledon in the 1960s covering the famous English tournament for UPI. One morning a little old lady approached him.

'Excuse me, sir. Are you Adrian Quist [a famous Australian tennis player of the 1930s]?'

'Me? Adrian Quist?' roared Dewhurst, bristling. 'Madam, I'll have you know it's only 10 a.m. How could I possibly be Adrian Quist?' The little old lady wandered away quite confused.

'Our Indian rubber keeper Ron Corry told everyone not to worry, that he would save the penalty. Incredibly, he did.'

22. SO NEAR, YET SO FAR

JOE VLASITS WAS determined nothing was going to be left to chance when we tried for a place in the 1970 World Cup finals in Mexico.

We had a series of 'friendlies' against one of our prospective opponents, Japan, in 1968 and then settled down for a marathon year in 1969. Of course, FIFA did us no favours. To make the finals we had to play nine international matches in the space of a few short months all around the world. There was one reason for this situation, sporting politics. It wasn't made any easier by the fact that our players were virtually all amateurs, unless you count the pittance the Australian Soccer Federation paid them. The rest of the countries that made the finals had teams of players that were nearly all well-paid professionals.

To tune us up for the qualifiers we had a three-match series of friendlies against Greece. We won 1–0 in front of 30,000 fans at the Sydney Cricket Ground in July 1969. We then drew 2–all in a vicious encounter at the Exhibition Ground in Brisbane where one of the Greek players was sent off and the Greek coach kept running on to the pitch only to be sent packing by the referee. The Aussies showed considerable restraint despite being kicked and punched. We were down 2–0 at one stage and Joe made an impassioned speech at half-time that stirred everyone up. Our blokes were disappointing in the third encounter in Melbourne, going down 2–0, failing to finish many promising moves.

In early October it was off to the South Korean capital of Seoul for a round robin against the home side and Japan (both good teams). The xenophobic South Korean crowd was the most hostile I have ever seen or heard. I have to admit that on future trips I found the crowds much more sportsman-like, but on this occasion the spectators were really nasty. We won through but not before some more drama. We had to win or draw the last match against South Korea. The team played well but the referee did us no favours. It may sound paranoid, but playing in Asia in those days was really hazardous. I wondered whether the ref was intimidated by the crowd. He disallowed a goal by Johnny Warren for an offside that for the life of me wasn't. Then the ref gave them a penalty they didn't deserve.

When that happened I was sure it was all over for us, but our keeper Ron Corry told everyone not to worry, he would save the penalty. Incredibly, he did. Ron developed quite a reputation for saving goals.

WE HAD A couple of weeks back home and then it was off to play Rhodesia in Lorenco Marques (now called Maputo), the capital of Mozambique when that country was still under Portuguese rule. Because of political problems associated with apartheid in South Africa and perceived similar racial problems in neighbouring Rhodesia (now Zimbabwe), South Korea had banned the Rhodesians from playing in Seoul in the qualifying tournament. Now, as winners, we had to play Rhodesia. The same predicament meant we had to play the two matches, so-called home and away, in neighbouring Mozambique. There was no racial conflict in the Rhodesian team that was made up of three white and eight black players, all of whom got on very well together. We managed to win after a third and deciding match (see *Chapter 27, My Friend the Witch Doctor*) and then had to fly to Israel for the first of the final two playoffs.

Once again we were stuffed up.

We arrived in the South African city of Johannesburg en route to Mozambique only to find the airline had cancelled some of our seats. So nearly half the team couldn't travel on immediately. Joe put me in charge of those players left behind. By the time we found our hotel accommodation it was fairly late and we headed off for bed. In the morning I had to find a ground where the team could train after lunch.

At 5 a.m. we were all woken by the hotel switchboard. The lady on the switch said we had ordered an early morning wake-up call. It was a ghastly hour but since we were all awake I decided to make the best of it by taking the blokes on a training run through the city streets. I had no idea where we were going but off we went in the dark. When we arrived back at our hotel a couple of hours later, we were met by distressed members of the hotel management. Worried about our safety, they had called the police. Nobody, but nobody, walked or ran through the area we had nominated at that time of day. The chances of being murdered, especially if you were white, were too great.

I wasn't game to tell Joe about that when we finally caught up with him.

The flight out of South Africa on our return also presented a problem. Because of the apartheid policy every surrounding country had banned any aircraft that flew to or from South Africa from using their air space. So our plane had to take a wide berth west of the African continent to Portugal, then to Rome and on to Athens before flying into Tel Aviv. We finally arrived, a very tired team, about 24 hours before we had to play Israel.

Under the circumstances of playing away, and considering how good a team Israel had, a loss 1–0 to them (with Corry saving another penalty and several booming shots from the Israeli strikers) was not too bad a result. When we arrived back home, Uncle Joe had visions of keeping the team together in camp in Sydney to prepare for the vital next game one week later. Unbelievably, with a World Cup finals spot in the offing, the Federation bosses refused his request. Joe was devastated. He felt betrayed, but all his pleading made no difference. He couldn't budge them. Before a capacity crowd of 32,500 at the old Sydney Sports Ground (on the site of what is now the Sydney Football Stadium) a 1–1 result with a late goal to John Watkiss was not sufficient.

Our marathon performance had been to no avail.

A SHAMEFUL DECISION

With no help from the Australian Soccer Federation hierarchy, Uncle Joe Vlasits got the Australian team to within a whisker of making the 1970 World Cup finals. For his Herculean efforts he was unceremoniously dumped. The decision to sack him says a lot more about soccer's officials than it does about Joe.

SO NEAR, YET SO FAR | 159

Look at his impressive record with the Australian side: 24 games, 14 wins and only 3 losses in full internationals, plus several other wins against teams on tour.

5 Nov, 1967	New Zealand Won 5-3	Saigon
7 Nov, 1967	South Vietnam Won 1-0	Saigon
11 Nov, 1967	Singapore Won 5-1	Saigon
12 Nov, 1967	Malaysia Won 1-0	Saigon
14 Nov, 1967	South Korea Won 3-2	Saigon
17 Nov, 1967	Indonesia Won 2-0	Jakarta
19 Nov, 1967	Indonesia Won 3-1	Jakarta
21 Nov, 1967	Singapore Won 6-1	Singapore
26 Nov, 1967	Malaysia Won 4-0	Kuala Lumpur
30 Mar, 1968	Japan Drawn 2-2	Sydney
31 Mar, 1968	Japan Won 3-1	Melbourne
4 Apr, 1968	Japan Lost 1-3	Adelaide
19 July, 1969	Greece Won 1-0	Sydney
23 July, 1969	Greece Drawn 2-2	Brisbane
26 July, 1969	Greece Lost 0-2	Melbourne
10 Oct, 1969	Japan *Won 3-1	Seoul
14 Oct, 1969	South Korea *Won 2-1	Seoul
16 Oct, 1969	Japan *Drawn 1-1	Seoul
20 Oct, 1969	South Korea *Drawn 1-1	Seoul
23 Nov, 1969	Rhodesia *Drawn 1-1	Lorenco Marques
27 Nov, 1969	Rhodesia *Drawn 0-0	Lorenco Marques
29 Nov, 1969	Rhodesia *Won 3-1	Lorenco Marques
4 Dec, 1969	Israel *Lost 0-1	Tel Aviv
14 Dec, 1969	Israel *Drawn 1-1	Sydney

* *World Cup qualifiers*

(Vlasits' Australian sides also beat Combined Services 8-1 at Singapore in 1967, and Kowloon Bus Company 8-1 and South Vietnam Army 1-0 in 1970)

'The security chief jumped out of our bus, grabbed the man and wrenched him out of his car. He then clouted him violently across the head.'

23. A TOUGH ROAD TO GERMANY

AUSTRALIA HAS ONLY qualified for the World Cup finals on one occasion — in West Germany in 1974. It was quite a feat as only 16 nations used to qualify in those days, half as many as make the final cut today. How Australia, under coach Rale Rasic, qualified to get to Germany is a story in itself.

Rasic came from his native Yugoslavia to Melbourne in 1962 and played at fullback for the JUST team, returned to Belgrade to obtain a physical education degree and then came back to Australia. He played in the winning Ampol Cup team and also for Victoria but plagued by injury he retired at the age of just 29 and took to coaching the Footscray-JUST team (as it had become known) in 1967. Two years later his team won the Victorian League Championship and he took over as coach of the Victorian team. He also won the national title with the Victorian Youth team. In 1971 he moved to Sydney to coach St George–Budapest, which that year won the grandfinal in the top four play-offs, followed by a most successful tour of Japan.

I first met Rale in 1969 when he attended the coaching course that Joe Vlasits, Denis Adrigan and I had organised at Epping in Sydney. He was very pleasant, good-looking and obviously very ambitious — nothing wrong with that, you have to be if you ever want to get anywhere. I nicknamed him 'Big Tree', telling him the story Don Bradman had told me about jealousy (the shade of the big tree of fame).

In 1970 he was appointed Australian coach to succeed Joe Vlasits. I thought that was a good decision, although he was only 34 and there were many rumblings about his youth and inexperience. He took the team on the highly ambitious World tour, starting in Noumea and playing 15 games in 10 different countries in five weeks, with some outstanding results including wins against Iran, Israel and Greece (the latter with the inevitable riot, but this time the crowd was trying to kill their own players, screaming in Greek 'Shame, Shame'). By the time we reached Mexico, it was a very tired soccer team, as they were after all only part-time players, and we were playing a good team at high altitude. We lost 3–0 with Ray Richards, one of our greatest and toughest mid-field players and definitely one of our greatest characters, being sent off. He had been fouled a couple of times by the Mexican captain, and the last time Ray fell on the ball. That was a funny sight as Ray hurled the ball, he had the most powerful throw, in the guy's face, and walked off with the referee desperately blowing his whistle demanding he return to be formally sent off. Amid the whistling and booing, Ray was pelted with all sorts of things, including cushions and oranges. He picked up one of the oranges and threw it back into the crowd. Another good shot.

OUR ROAD TO the finals began with a tournament in Australasia involving the Socceroos, New Zealand, Iraq and Indonesia. The Iraqis started as hot favourites, but as every punter knows, the bookmakers are not always right. Our first game was against New Zealand in Auckland. Outplayed, we were lucky to escape with a 1–1 draw. Australia later drew again with our Trans-Tasman neighbours in Sydney (this time 3–3). We advanced to the next round after an outstanding 3–1 victory and a 0–0 draw against Iraq and two victories over Indonesia (2–1 and 6–0). The second encounter with Indonesia at the Sydney Sports Ground was a real pressure match, as Iraq had beaten the New Zealanders 4–0 earlier in the afternoon at the same arena to put them one point ahead of us. The result against Indonesia was never in doubt from the moment that Jim Mackay scored Australia's first goal after just three minutes.

This meant we to had play off, home and away, with Iran. Australia would be without the rugged Manfred Schaefer who was recovering after surgery on a torn cartilage, but the Iranians were also hard hit by the absence of mid-fielder Ali Parvin. He was just 17 at the time but already showing the skills that would make him a legend in Iranian football, with 82 international caps. Parvin had suffered a leg injury in a warm-up friendly in New Zealand.

We played very well against the Iranians in Sydney in front of a crowd of almost 31,000, winning 3–0. We then travelled with them in the same plane to Teheran for the return match six days later. The Iranians were very apprehensive, as it turned out, for very good reasons.

The plane arrived just before dawn. A massive, hostile and intimidating crowd was waiting. Johnny Warren and I decided to wander out of the airport precincts to see what the commotion was all about. What a sight awaited us! Cyclone fencing had been put up around the entrance and hundreds of people in the crowd were trying to climb over it. As they clambered up the fence a small army of police was belting their hands producing enough broken fingers to discourage the climbers from trying again. What surprised us was that they weren't screaming for Australian blood, but for the blood of their own team. That's how angry they were about the Sydney defeat.

As a stunningly beautiful dawn was breaking over Teheran both teams were quickly whisked away in buses from the back of the airport in an attempt to get away from the fanatical fans. However, there was a huge monument to the Shah of Iran (he and it had not yet been toppled) at a roundabout on the way to the centre of the city. More of this ferocious Iranian welcoming committee had gathered at the roundabout, but were in cars this time. The buses drove straight through the middle of the roundabout with the cars taking up the chase in a long line behind us.

We had quite a few security men on our bus, all hardened officers from the much-feared Iranian secret police, the Savak, who were tough, ruthless and uncaring. When we reached our hotel barricades were hastily thrown up behind the buses. The Savak raced into the hotel, grabbed everyone unlucky enough to be in the foyer, including relatives of their own team, and unceremoniously dumped them into the street. Not one of them was willing to protest about their treatment.

The Iranians had another trick to play. We had brought with us a large consignment of meat from Sydney, but it was left out in the hot Iranian sun and no amount of pleading could permit its release for three days. It was not much use to anyone after that.

WE PLAYED IRAN in front of 80,000 ear-shattering fans at the new Aryamehr Stadium amid the tightest security imaginable. There was even a tank parked just outside the gates. It was hot, awfully hot, and awfully humid and we were playing at high altitude. The fans kept saluting with four fingers, suggesting that was how many goals their team would score. The fanatical crowd made so much noise that the players could not communicate with each other.

Never in all my years have I seen a team play like the Iranians did for that first half. With Parvin back in action and playing wonderfully in the mid-field, they kept running at us at a furious pace in wave after wave, at times with a three-man overlap, and we were scrambling just to contain them. After a quarter of an hour, the Soviet referee found a penalty to give against us. No one else at the ground seemed to understand what it was for, but I suppose it did ensure his physical survival at the end of the game. At half-time the score was 2–0 to them and our original three-goal advantage was being whittled away.

Rasic made two important clever switches. Our striker, Noddy Alston, was being kicked to death by the two large Iranian defenders and Noddy wasn't able to get a shot in. At half-time, Max Tolson was brought on in his place. Max told me afterwards that Rasic had warned him the two defenders would be trying to kick the shit out of him, too, but that didn't worry Max, for the tougher it was the more he revelled in it. He took both defenders on using their own tactics plus a few of his own, demolishing them both.

The other move came during the second half when Johnny Warren was replaced by Jim Rooney. The Iranians were at last visibly tiring and Jim was a genius for holding the ball, thus denying the Iranians possession, despite their flying boots and elbows. When the final whistle blew with the score remaining 2–0 the Socceroos had pulled off what had seemed, at one stage, an almost impossible victory.

WE HAD THE chief Savak man with us in the bus on the way back to our hotel. He had been trained in America by the CIA and spoke perfect English with an American accent. He was a big, fit man who was surprisingly friendly, quite charming even.

Suddenly a car drove up level with our bus and the driver of the car leant out the window to say something, doubtless pointing out, not in polite language, how fortunate we had been to win through. I didn't think anyone could hear him above the din, but our Savak man leapt up and ordered the bus driver to cross over into the other lane and pull up in front of the car. The security chief jumped out of our bus, grabbed the man and wrenched him out of his car. He then clouted him violently across the head with some sort of waddy before throwing him unconscious and bleeding onto the road. Finally he ripped the keys from the car's ignition, so no one else could drive, got back in the bus and waved the driver on. It all happened in the wink of an eye. The Savak boss sat down next to me and continued chatting as though nothing had happened. No wonder Savak were feared and loathed.

DID THAT GET us to the World Cup Finals? No way, for there were still two matches, home and away, to be played against South Korea to decide who went to Germany. More than 32,000 fans turned up at the Sydney Sports Ground to cheer us on in the first leg, but the Socceroos were disappointing, and gave a lacklustre display, especially in the midfield. Our only chance to score fell to Noddy Alston, 32 minutes into the game, but his shot drifted wide. Goalkeeper Jim Fraser, recently recovered from a bad back injury to play a blinder, made a couple of spectacular saves of shots that could have given the Koreans victory. The game ended in a nil–all draw.

A fortnight later in Seoul the Socceroos faced their greatest test. The balmy spring weather of Sydney was long forgotten in the freezing temperatures of Seoul. On the morning of the match, light snow fell on the Municipal Stadium. The South Koreans began with a real blitzkrieg and after half an hour were two goals in front. The situation looked ominous for Australia. The Socceroos pulled one goal back almost immediately with a classic header from striker Branko Buljevic. A long throw-in from Ray Richards found Ray Baartz, Australia's most capped player at that time, in the centre of the penalty area and he banged in the equaliser. The Socceroos' spirits visibly lifted as they went after the winning goal. A shot from Atti Abonyi narrowly slipped over the crossbar, Buljevic banged one into the outside of the net and a boomer from Peter Wilson bounced of one of the uprights. Time eventually ran out. With a 2–all draw, it was off to Hong Kong where two days later the spot in the World Cup finals would be decided.

IT WAS ANOTHER change in weather, this time to almost 100 per cent humidity. Although there was torrential rain before the game, the ground's superb drainage enabled the clash to go ahead as scheduled.

There were many close calls that with luck could have given Australia goals — a Buljevic header, then a Buljevic drive from 20 metres out and a mix up between him and Baartz that resulted in a fluffed shot at goal.

Half-time: 0–0.

In the 70th minute Australia's luck changed for the better. They received an indirect free kick. Richards' shot was headed back downfield. Rooney was 'Jimmy on the Spot' chipping it back to expatriate Scot Jim Mackay, who in turn, surged towards the goal before hammering a right foot kick from 35 metres out into the top left-hand corner of the net. The shot was unstoppable.

Australia missed with a couple of other attempts, but it didn't matter — even if the countdown to the final whistle was almost unbearable for those of us on the bench. Mackay's 'golden goal' had won the Socceroos a place in the World Cup finals.

'A belter wasn't it!' smiled Mackay. 'The second I hit it I knew it was going all the way.'

The guys chaired Rasic, captain Wilson and hero Mackay off the pitch, with Mackay waving that wonderful right boot of his like an Olympic torch. That night the players drank champagne from the boot.

We were the centre of attention at Sydney Airport when we returned triumphant. Photographers jostled to take photos of Jim, with his three-year-old son Malcolm in one arm and waving the boot with the other.

'It's not going to a museum,' he told reporters. 'And I'm not selling it either. I'm keeping it for Malcolm. Kids all over the country can now look at the Australian Soccer team with pride and tell their dads they want to play the game.' (Since Jim's death, Malcolm has come to the team's reunions.)

Soon we would be off to Germany to do battle.

Well, most of us would. To soccer's eternal shame Ray Baartz never made it onto the pitch in the finals shoot-out.

'Did Garisto get punished? Not a chance. They feted him as a hero and FIFA was too weak to do anything about what had happened.'

24. A SPORTING TRAGEDY

APRIL 27 1974. Mark it down as a day of infamy in Australian sporting history. Not because of what any of our sporting stars did, but for what a visiting player inflicted on one of our greatest athletes. I cannot call the culprit a sportsman. For there was nothing sporting about what was done to Ray Baartz at the Sydney Cricket Ground that day.

Baartz was Australia's most successful international soccer star. Newcastle born and bred, he had spent two years in England learning his trade as an apprentice at Manchester United under the great tutor, Matt Busby. Just when the world was beckoning, Baartz returned home because he was homesick. He was soon the toast of the Australian soccer world as a striker with the Sydney club Hakoah and it was only a matter of time before he was called into the Socceroo squad. There he stayed from 1967 to 1974, scoring 21 goals in his then record 59 appearances.

What happened to Ray Baartz at the Sydney Cricket Ground that April day turned out to be, not only a sporting tragedy, a personal tragedy for this very amiable sportsman who always played the game fairly and never had a bad word to say about anyone.

The Socceroos were fine-tuning their side in preparation for the World Cup finals. Among the so-called 'friendlies' were two against another Cup final qualifier, Uruguay. On Anzac Day Australia had drawn nil–all with the visitors in Melbourne. The Uruguayans did not like any of it. The game was incredibly rough with iron-man Manfred Schaefer injured and unable to finish.

The mood of the Uruguayan players was no different in the second encounter in Sydney two days later. Before the game they demanded we drop Gary Manuel, who had stood up to their rough-house tactics in Melbourne. We dismissed the Uruguayan ultimatum out of hand. What they didn't know was that Manuel wasn't going to play anyway because he had injured an ankle in the first encounter, the injury forcing his replacement in the 62nd minute.

It was 'anything goes' from the kick-off in Sydney. The visitors, unaccustomed to being held, became more and more frustrated. On the other hand Australia was playing some really good football. Just on the hour, Baartz scored and we went on to win 2–0.

But behind the play, with 15 minutes to go, defender, Luis Garisto, hit Baartz with the side of his palm in a kind of karate chop aimed upwards and catching him just under the jaw. Baartz went down like a sack of potatoes. Don Campbell, who subsequently went on to become one of our top referees, was controlling his first match and didn't see the incident, but his linesman did! As Don went to send off Garisto, the Uruguayans milled around him, jostling and man-handling him in a dreadful display of high dudgeon and lousy sportsmanship (to say the least). This disgraceful exhibition went on for quite some time.

While I was tending to Ray, who was lying very groggy on the ground, I witnessed an astounding incident. The Uruguayan captain took their striker Fernando Morena around behind the referee and gave him a swift hard clout on the mouth. Morena was then dragged back in front of referee Campbell, and his bleeding lip was triumphantly shown, with the captain saying that Ray had hit him and Garisto had run in to help his team-mate. Look at the damage Baartz had caused the Uruguayans shouted. Don was not having a bar of that and was finally able to persuade Garisto he had to leave the field, sent off on a charge of violent conduct. Ray staggered to his feet and said he could continue playing, but he was clearly unwell.

More drama followed. Almost immediately Morena put the ball in the back of the net. The referee was on the spot and ruled it was a handball. If the Uruguayans were going on like pork chops earlier, there was no stopping them now. They were baying for blood. Luckily, the game ended soon after that, but on a very sour note.

Did Garisto get punished? Not a chance. They feted him as a hero and FIFA was too weak to do anything about what had happened.

Soon after the match, Ray said he was having headaches and felt weak down one side, like he'd had a stroke. He was rushed to Royal North Shore Hospital where tests that night showed that the artery on the right side supplying blood to the brain had been torn by the karate blow and was blocked. His treatment was complete hospital rest and close observation.

Ray Baartz gradually improved, but never played football again. At the age of 27 the career of one of the best and fairest players Australia has ever seen had been brought to an end by a foul blow from an unrepentant miscreant.

The brilliance of Baartz was sorely missed in Germany, even though he travelled with us on our campaign to provide moral support.

Baartz never returned to the scene of this awful incident until late 2003, just before the 30th anniversary of the Socceroos' successful World Cup qualification. Although he never played again, he changed his focus and carved out a successful business career. 'You can't let something like that rule you,' he said. 'I just got on with my life.'

JOKE BACKFIRES

We had two warm-up matches on the way to Germany, beating Indonesia 2–1 in Jakarta, watched by some 62,000 fans. It cost us dearly as Col Curran injured a knee ligament and only through his sheer determination and lots of exercise in pools did we have him ready to play in Germany.

We then flew into Tel Aviv for a match in Israel and security was really tight. On the way there we were ribbing Ray Richards about his dark appearance and big moustache. We told him he looked just like a terrorist and would have trouble getting in. We didn't expect that as soon as we landed he would disappear — he was indeed grabbed by the security police as a suspected terrorist. It turned out that he had a strange resemblance to a wanted man. His cause may not have been helped by some of his team-mates agreeing with the police that he was the man they were after. He needed help from the Israeli soccer officials before he was eventually released some time later.

A SPORTING TRAGEDY | 169

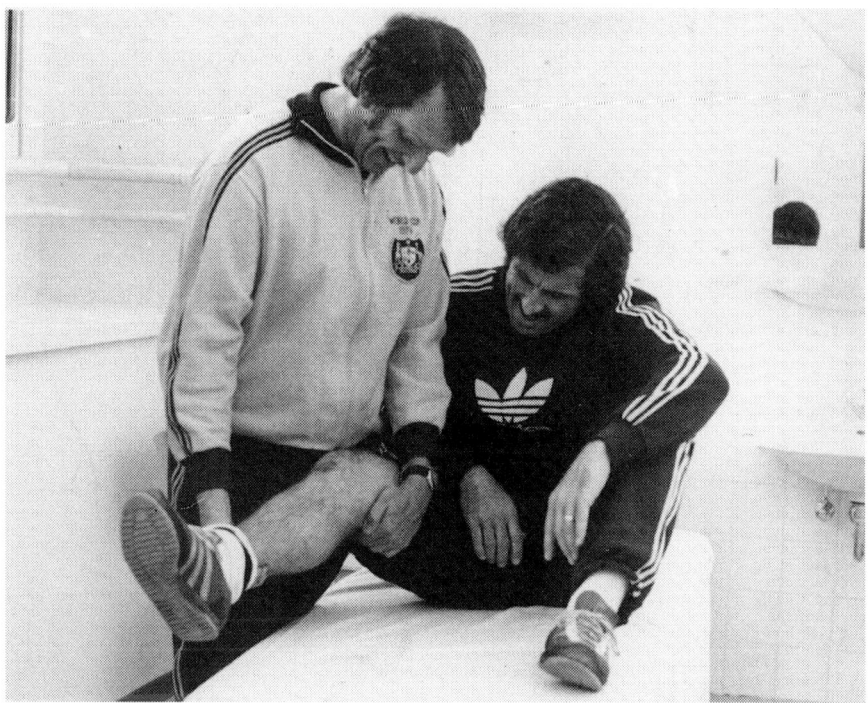

Doing my job. Attending to Australian soccer great, Ray Richards.
BRIAN CORRIGAN'S COLLECTION

Ray was a tough, uncompromising mid-field player who gave his all for his adopted country from the time he was first picked in 1967. His greatest moment surely came in 1972 when the famous Brazilian club Santos toured with Pele, the greatest soccer player of all time. Coach Rale Rasic gave him strict instructions he was not to foul Pele, an instruction which ran counter to all Ray's natural instincts. He marked Pele tight but fairly and Pele rarely got away from him, didn't score and Ray only fouled him once and that might have been a genuine mistake. Pele was most impressed and said that Ray was one of the best he had ever played against. It was very high praise.

This game was played at the Sydney Sports Ground before a packed crowd. Before kick-off there was high drama and the start was delayed for a long time with the crowd getting increasingly restless. Santos had demanded that the team be paid in American dollars. The problem was that not enough American dollars could be found on a weekend. Cheques? Not good enough. They could have the gate takings. Not good enough. Two Australian millionaires gave their personal guarantees.

Not good enough. Santos threatened they would take their team home. Imagine the riot that would have caused. In the end the money was found because officials managed to persuade a bank to come to the rescue.

We lost 2-1 to a determined Israel in Tel Aviv when Rasic was away watching the East German team in Leipzig. We were due to play a second match against the Israelis, two days later in Jerusalem, but the field had pieces of broken glass in it. I ruled it impossible to play on because of the risk of injury to our stars. That decision almost caused a riot, but the players' wellbeing was paramount.

'It did a power of good to see the German team coming off at half-time with the score 0-0, their heads down, arguing among themselves.'

25. IN THE MAJOR LEAGUE

D-DAY WAS FAST approaching. We had a short, pleasant stay at Zug in Switzerland in early June 1974, winning matches against local teams St Gallen, Young Boys and Neuchatel to ready us for the big encounters ahead.

Then it was on to our World Cup 'home' at Oschenzoll, just outside Hamburg. This had many advantages for it was the training ground for the Hamburg football club with many beautifully kept pitches on which to train. Also, the quarters, accommodation and food were of a very high standard, a novel experience for us.

What was not so good was the incredibly strict security with armed guards and police vans everywhere. The Germans obviously did not want a repeat of the fiasco of the terrorist attacks of the Munich Olympics two years before. But they definitely carried the security a bit too far, as the players' friends and visitors from Australia quickly discovered. For all that, quite amazingly, the security was concentrated at the front and sides of the building, while at the back, where all the open training fields were located, there was none. I used to look out my window at night and muse how a terrorist had only to cross the fields and they were in my room.

The other problem was boredom, as all the players had to do was train morning and afternoon, and had to rest for the remainder of the day. They did have television and movies, but they were in German. The only one who understood a word of German was Manfred Schaefer. In addition to all of this the players were only allowed out to go to official functions and not drink. Ho hum!! Boredom was the direct cause of the loss of our striker Max Tolson. He was kicking a ball against the wall and very nearly severed his toe on the sharp edge of a radiator. We had to sew it up in the middle of the night and he could not play in the finals. Rasic was furious.

But for the Socceroos, almost unknown back in Australia, being in Germany was a novel experience. Wherever we travelled on the team bus, people along the way would stand on the footpaths and cheer for us enthusiastically. One reason may have been that Schaefer was in our team. He had been born in East Germany and quickly became a crowd favourite. The Germans called him 'The Milkman' because that was his job back in Sydney.

AUSTRALIA'S GROUP CONSISTED of East Germany, West Germany and Chile. The first game at the Volksparkstadion in Hamburg was against East Germany, which was quite a good team at that time. They started at a predictably fast rate for they really believed they would win easily against us. Our instructions were to contain them as much as possible, which we were doing extremely well. It did a power of good to see the East German team coming off at half-time with the score 0–0, their heads down, arguing among themselves. More than that, the West German crowd had turned against them, possibly for the ideological reasons of East versus West and they were cheering for us.

Early in the second-half, the East Germans made a break down the right. The Australians held back waiting for what seemed like an obvious offside to be whistled up. It didn't come. The ball ricocheted off Col Curran for an own goal and we were down 1–0.

From then on, the Australians played magnificently as they took the attack to the East Germans, missing a goal by a whisker when one shot hit the post. The inevitable happened — the defence was left open at the back and they scored another goal.

Everyone who had watched the Socceroos' great fight had tremendous admiration for such a gutsy, hard-running performance and how we'd fought back against the odds. Well, everyone except our coach, who wanted a draw. With a touch of luck we would have had it.

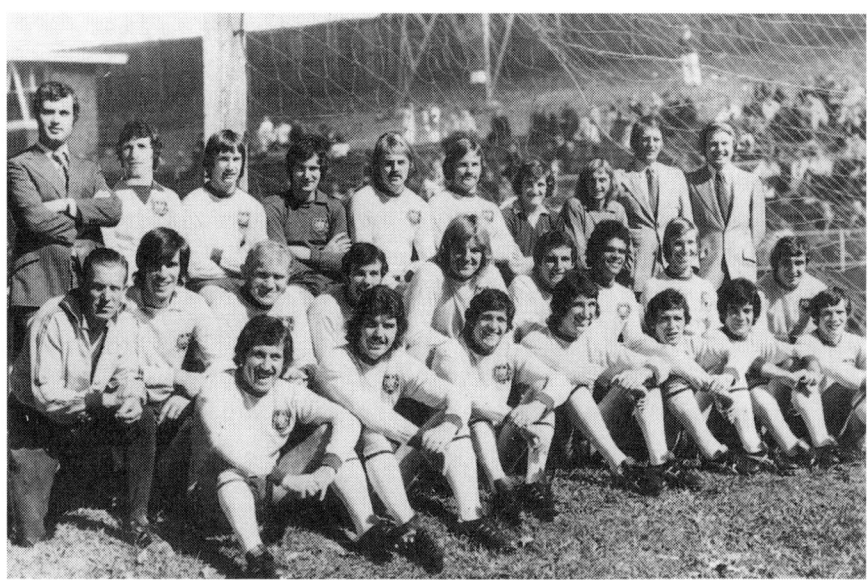
Training camp, Sydney 1973. (BRIAN CORRIGAN'S COLLECTION)

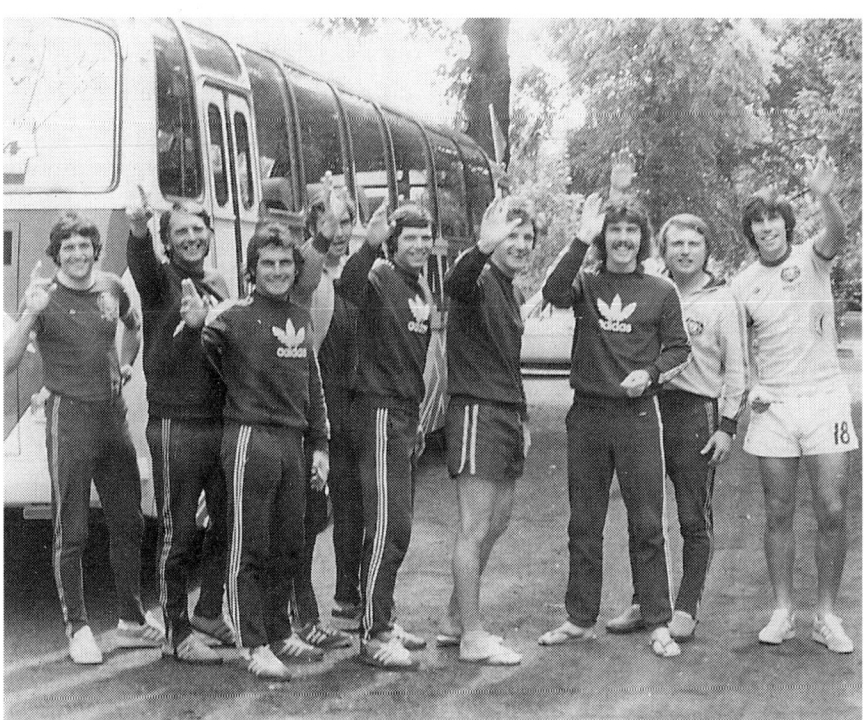
A happy group catching the team bus in Hamburg in 1974.
(BRIAN CORRIGAN'S COLLECTION)

There was no doubt that we didn't stand a chance against West Germany, who were pre-tournament favourites and ultimately went on to win the World Cup final (against The Netherlands). The West Germans had not played particularly well in their first game, against Chile, but they won 3–0 against the Socceroos and even then were not often playing, really flat out. Franz Beckenbauer, the captain and one of the all-time greats of the game, didn't seem particularly interested at all, a fact the crowd quickly picked up on and roundly booed and whistled him. Again, for a different reason, the West German crowd was barracking for us. Unbelievable! Beckenbauer's reply was to show them his bared buttocks. Not a pretty sight. This performance prompted even more whistling.

It was on to Berlin for our last game against Chile in the Olympic Stadium built by the Nazis for the 1936 Olympics. You could still see bullet holes from the World War II battle for Berlin in 1945 when the Russians finally overran the city. It had started to rain a bit before the match, but at half-time it suddenly became a deluge.

Again we had tight security. Our security man could have been a clone of the Savak man in Iran. Yet he seemed a nice guy; tough, CIA-trained. He told me that they were on special alert because they had been warned there would be a demonstration by Chilean students protesting against the brutal right-wing regime of Augusto Pinochet that had, the year before, thrown out the democratically-elected government of socialist Salvador Allende.

The rain was so heavy that it was difficult to see the other side of the ground and the security men were forced to take refuge under the stand. At that moment, the Chilean students, waving their flags and protest banners, leapt over the fence and started running across the ground. They were quickly rounded up by the security men and taken under the stand where they were given a ferocious beating. Our chief security man was in tears, not because of what was happening to the poor students, because he had tried so hard to prevent this happening. Now what would his superiors say? I can't say I had any sympathy for him.

The match turned into a farce as the ground was flooded and nobody could control the ball. Kick the ball and it would just stop dead in a puddle. Then the referee lost control of the game. Col Curran (has there ever been a better or gutsier left fullback play for Australia?) was carried off on a stretcher when the medial ligament of his knee was snapped in a late tackle.

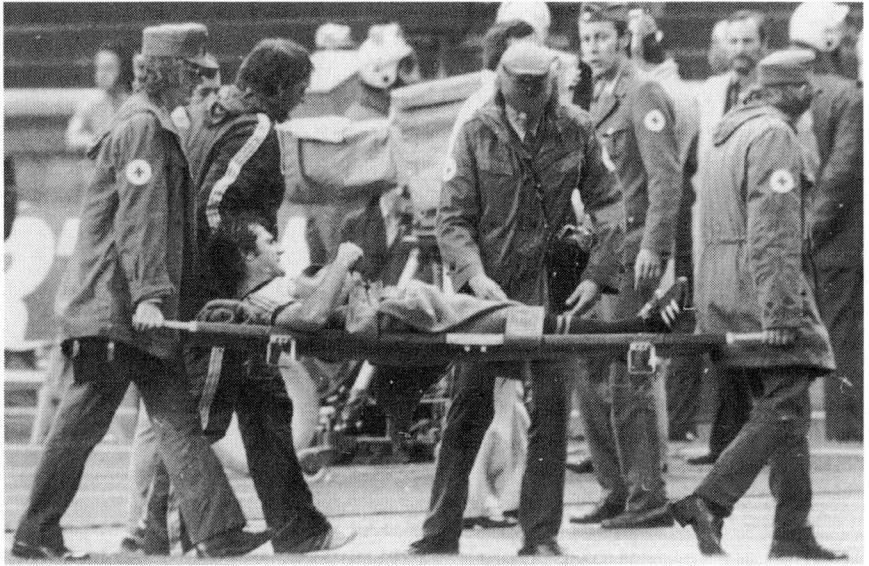

During our messy final game against Chile in Berlin — heavy rain, Chilean protesters invading the pitch — our fullback Col Curran snapped a ligament in his knee in a late tackle and had to be carried from the field. (BRIAN CORRIGAN'S COLLECTION)

In the 83rd minute the Chilean striker was fouled. While Ray Richards was, with great difficulty, trying to look innocent, the referee was handing a card to Manfred Schaefer, who was explaining, as sweetly as Manfred ever could, that it could not possibly have been him. The linesman called the referee over and told him to change his call and Ray ended up with a red card.

It made no difference. The referee eventually blew an end to the farce. And at nil–all Australia came away with its first (and to this day only) World Cup point.

THROUGHOUT THE WORLD Cup campaign, Rasic had his critics. Surprise, surprise, tell me what coach didn't. Some reckoned he was too abrasive. Rale's reply, 'I was a coach not a diplomat. If I were a diplomat we would never have qualified.' Many believed he played too defensively, especially when we were lucky to escape with those two draws against New Zealand in the preliminary matches. Rale was always supremely confident in his own ability. At the World Cup finals when any coach there for the first time, and especially one so young as he was, would be entitled to be overawed, he took to it as though he had been coaching World Cup teams all his life. He had one outstanding characteristic that may be shared with other coaches, but I am sure never to the degree Rale had, total recall for a game, what each player did or did not do or should have done at any particular time, and he still has this gift.

He had some monumental quarrels and arguments with ASF president Sir Arthur George over a whole range of matters, they were very different personalities. Rale had never been afraid to speak his mind and criticise the powers that be about the many things that he (and many other people, for that matter) thought was wrong with Australian soccer. Arthur introduced Rale to NSW Premier Robin Askin saying, 'He is a great coach, but he is also a son of a bitch.' I think Rale loved both assertions.

Some arguments came about because Rale was standing up for his team. There was a player's strike in camp just before the playoff against South Korea in Sydney in 1973. Rale demanded a meeting with Arthur to try to resolve the strike. Arthur said there was no money, walked out and drove off. Some players started packing. Game, Set and Match Point. Arthur turned his car around, the meeting became more amicable the second time and some (and I mean some) money was found. Game on, just in time!

When Rale returned home from the World Cup, things started to go very, very wrong. Some officials claimed he had become big-headed. 'I was a bit cocky,' Rasic admits. After all, he had threatened during the finals to resign when they were finished.

There was also a disagreement with Arthur to do with money. Whether it had been promised or not, there was nothing in writing, and Rale took that as proof that his criticisms of ASF incompetence were correct. He decided to take Arthur on and was reported to have said, 'Either you go or I go.' There could only be one winner in that confrontation. Rale went — sacked. The full story of that bitter time has never been published, as far as I am aware, but I am sure it will one day.

A golden opportunity to promote the game was lost and I often wonder just what could have become of it all if that 'clash of titans' had turned out differently.

Rasic continued to coach in Sydney, Melbourne and Adelaide — in total 312 matches for 122 wins, but things never seemed the same for him again after those halcyon World Cup days when anything and everything seemed possible for Australian soccer and its coach.

BRIBED TO WIN

During the preliminary matches in Australia's vain attempt to get to the 1978 World Cup finals in Argentina, I was the manager of our team with Jim Shoulder as the coach. After beating off Taiwan (3-0 and 2-1) and New Zealand (3-1 and 1-1), we were then drawn in a group with Iran, Kuwait, South Korea and Hong Kong. After losing two of our home matches (1-0 to Iran in Melbourne and 2-1 to Kuwait in Sydney) and winning two (3-0 over Hong Kong and 2-1 over South Korea) we headed off for the return legs. We drew 0-0 in Seoul against South Korea which put us in a perilous position. A 5-2 victory in Hong Kong helped revive our spirits a little for a do or die effort in Kuwait. In a spiteful game there, in which John Kosmina was sent off in the 56th minute, we lost 1-0. This meant that, for all intents and purposes, we were effectively out of the competition and we had no realistic chance of qualifying for the next World Cup.

The problem I faced as manager was whether or not you can be bribed to win. Yes, I did say bribed to win. Let me explain. After the game some of the local coaches who were Englishmen came around to tell me that the Kuwaitis would turn up to offer us a bribe, not a bribe to lose against Iran, but one to win against them. They said the Kuwaitis were getting in first as they were worried that when we reached Iran we would be given an even larger bribe by the locals to lose.

Sure enough, a sheik did arrive at our hotel to say that if we won the next game against Iran in Teheran we would be paid a huge sum of American dollars. I said thank you very much but there was no point for such largesse because Australians always played to win, whatever the circumstances. He insisted that I should think about it and he would come again later to give instructions about how it was to be arranged.

The money would have been a huge bonus for the players, infinitely more than they were getting from the Australian Soccer Federation. When the sheik turned up carrying his suitcase full of money, I told him that we were really not interested in his bribe, but would try as hard as we could against Iran. He looked at me in disbelief. We travelled to Teheran, nobody from Iran turned up to bribe us. We lost 1-0. I was left to wonder whether we should have accepted his bribe to win and if he would have turned up at our hotel in Teheran with his suitcase had we done so.

A different scenario on the same trip. We had scheduled a friendly against Singapore six days before the away game in Kuwait and when we arrived in Singapore we were repeatedly asked what the score in our game would turn out to be. More in an effort to keep them quiet than anything else, Jim Shoulder would hold up two fingers to signify a 2–0 win to us, but I did wonder if that might have been a mistake.

For the first half, the refereeing of the game was flawless, no one could have had any complaints. If we bowled one of them over the ref gave them a free kick. If they bowled one of our players over, he gave us a free kick. Just on half-time we scored our second goal to lead 2–0.

You could not imagine the change after half-time. The referee seemed determined that we would not score again. On one occasion I was left shaking my head when he missed an incident from which we should have received a penalty. There was no further score and we won 2–0. The local officials came up after the game and apologised (that was a first). They told us it was the last game of the referee's career and he had taken Jim's prediction of a 2–0 victory literally!

SECOND OPINION

CHARLIE YANKOS

One of the greatest soccer players in the history of the Australian game. He was capped 87 times for Australia (between 1985 and 1989) and captained the Socceroos 30 times, including their surge to the quarter-finals at the 1988 Seoul Olympics. In 2003 he was seconded to serve on an eight-person task force charged with planning the blueprint for a new national competition in Australia.

NOT THE RETIRING TYPE

SPORTSMEN AND WOMEN had complete faith in Brian Corrigan. He had a real knack of diagnosing what was wrong with you, and (usually) having an instant remedy that would have you back in action almost overnight. He had the ability to have you laughing when things looked black.

Brian's expertise was unbelievable. In my years with the Socceroos I had so many major injuries in the lead-up to important games: World

Cup qualifiers, the 1988 Olympics and so on. I would have resigned myself to not playing, to watching from the sidelines. Come hell or high water, Doc Corrigan would get me back on the paddock.

He understood a sportsman's psyche. We wanted to play. If your injury was life-threatening or could result in major permanent damage, he would say 'No!' to you playing, and you would respect his judgment and do what he said. Otherwise he would find a way to have you back in action.

I was plagued by a chronic injury, the degeneration of my pubic bone, throughout my career. I remember talking about it with Doc Corrigan.

'There's only one answer,' he said with a knowing nod of the head. 'You'll have to retire.'

My jaw dropped. Then he roared with laughter.

'Well, you should retire, but we'll see what we can do for you,' he laughed.

On another occasion I was at the Australian Institute of Sport (AIS) in Canberra undergoing my medicals for the 1988 Olympic team. Doc Corrigan wasn't involved in the check-up but passed me in the corridor as I came out after the examination. I had been worried because at the time I was in such pain I could hardly touch my toes.

'How d'ya go?' he asked.

'I passed,' I told him.

'Passed?' he roared. 'I know all about you. There is no way they could have passed you.'

'Keep your voice down,' I hissed.

And then he burst out laughing.

He was of immense value to Australia's Socceroos, as I suspect he was for all sporting stars. No matter which country we went to, he had either been there before or had known someone who had. He knew the conditions we would play under and the injuries we faced, either because of the tactics of our opponents or the state of the pitches on which the matches were played, and he had a remedy for each of those injuries.

You have to remember we were like an extended family, to many of us Brian Corrigan was a father figure. Even when we were in

Australia we trusted our lives to him. At one stage I played in a World Cup qualifier against Fiji in 1988 at Newcastle. We won 5–1 but there was an all-in brawl and I ended up with a badly smashed nose, the media dubbed the match the 'Battle of Newcastle'. When they said they were taking me to hospital I refused unless Doc Corrigan came with me. I wasn't going to let any other doctor do anything unless Brian gave the green light.

Such was the case when we were playing Israel in a World Cup qualifier in 1985 at Tel Aviv. Our goalie Terry Greedy had an awful eye injury, and he wouldn't go to hospital unless the Doc went with him. We were worried about Terry as he looked a real mess when he left the pitch. We won the match 2–1 and went back to our hotel. There was no sign of Terry and Brian and we were a bit apprehensive.

'They'll turn up,' said one of the blokes. So we went around the corner to a bar that had caught our eye. As we walked in there was a bruised and battered Terry and the Doc, each with a half-finished beer in front of them.

'You won, didn't you?' snapped Brian. 'Well, what kept ya!'

'You must never argue with someone who does not know what he is talking about.'

26. MASSAGING THE SPIRIT

OVER THE YEARS Australian soccer teams have been most fortunate with the physiotherapists that have looked after them. The first two I knew remain vividly etched in my mind. To highlight the international nature of soccer, one was an Italian and the other a Dutchman — Lou Lazzari and Peter van Ryn. They differed in every way you could ever imagine.

Lou was real giant of a man with huge hands (great for massaging), a shock of white hair and a face that smiled easily and often. When we were in Vietnam the locals, who as a race were so much smaller than him, were genuinely in awe of Lou. They called him the 'Gentle Giant'. When we marched in the opening ceremony for the tournament we were playing in, all the cheering was for Lou.

He had a passionate love of football and the players whom he called 'my boys' and would do anything for them or the coach Joe Vlasits. Kind, courteous, dignified, untiring, at peace with himself and the world, Lou handed out his homespun advice as he listened to all their problems like the father-figure he became to them. He really believed his boys could do no wrong (I knew better). He could never see anything wrong in anyone or anything.

I remember how Lou took me aside one day when some pompous official was arguing with me. The more the official argued the hotter I got under the collar.

'Doctor,' Lou said in his soft voice. 'You must never argue with someone who does not know what he is talking about.' That particular piece of advice has stuck firmly in my mind ever since. Down to earth advice that would serve anyone, anywhere very well.

Lou's other love was his family. In Melbourne he would have me around to the family lunch, lots of Italian food and wine, and you could feel how proud he was of his wife and boys. The boys have all done well in life.

He retired from his soccer job in early 1970. At the time I was quite surprised to hear of his decision for he could have kept the job for as long as he wished.

Next time the team was in Melbourne he phoned to ask if he could come around to see me as he had a special request. Sure, Lou. The request was that I would take him around and introduce him to all the players.

'What are you talking about? You know them all better than I do!'

'Well, there may be a few new ones I may not have met, but I want you to introduce me to everyone.'

It wasn't true, but I thought I'd humour him and around the hotel we went. We'd knock on a player's door and when he answered I would introduce him to Mr Lou Lazzari, the player would look at me as if I had gone soft in the head (or even softer than usual). But Lou seemed happy. When we arrived back in my room he had tears in his eyes and he wrapped his huge hands around mine and said how grateful he was and how much I had done for him. As he left, he turned and said, 'Goodbye doctor.' I suddenly realised he had something wrong with him. This had been a charade for him, a way to say goodbye to his boys. It was true, Lou was dying. He said nothing that day and he died not long afterwards, very much missed.

WHAT A STARK contrast our next physio was!! Peter van Ryn was small, dark, restless, irascible, impatient to a degree, mischievous, couldn't stop still, stop talking, or stop swearing. I had met him some time before when he was working for the Hakoah club in Sydney and he talked then about how much he loved his soccer. So he seemed a good candidate for the job when Lou retired.

His first time with the team was a world trip in 1970 with Rale Rasic as coach. Our first game was in Noumea and Peter was even more excitable than usual. He kept walking around at the back of our bench, swearing about everyone from the referee down and giving his opinion about how each player was doing things wrong. The reserves sitting on the bench soon got thoroughly sick of his ranting and told him to shut up —that's a polite way of putting it. This made no difference to Peter. Finally, they had had enough. They picked Peter up and deposited him in his physio box just behind the corner flag, telling him not to move.

'That's better,' they said. 'At last we can hear ourselves think'.

There were rumblings about how he would have to be sent home because the players wouldn't be able to put up with him for a whole tour. Next thing there was this voice behind them. Peter was back swearing away about everything. It took a great deal to get everyone to settle down and I kept reassuring them that he would improve, even though I did have my doubts. And he did, at least he became a bit more manageable.

As the tour progressed things changed. He got less excitable and they got more used to him. What a funny character he turned out to be. By the time the long tour was over he had become an integral part of the team. The players realised his heart was in the right place. He would do anything for them and worked very hard. In the end they all loved him.

He particularly enjoyed going to Indonesia. In the past he had done a favour for some Indonesian army general and as soon as Peter arrived everything was laid on for him. It was a bit different on one occasion when we visited China. Accommodation was very tight and I drew the short straw — I had to room with him for the duration of the tour. It was a real problem as he hardly ever slept and preferred to talk all night. Worse things followed in one hotel when we found there was only one double bed in our room. We eyed each other suspiciously and I knew that there would be no sleep that night.

Peter did talk all that night, but what he told me was spellbinding. He told me lots of tales about how he had worked for the Resistance in Holland during World War II and spent much time in hiding as he was being tracked down by the Nazis. I had a new perspective on him.

A terrifying riot broke out after we had won 2–0 in a match against the South Vietnam Under-23s at Saigon in 1972. The reason it started was probably that we had played too vigorously. The reason didn't matter much for the petrified players and officials who had to huddle in the middle of the ground while being pelted with bottles and rocks. Kerosene was also thrown at us, some of it getting in the eye of my great friend Tom Patrick causing him intense pain and blindness, gratefully only temporarily. In the meantime the dressing shed was thoroughly demolished. The army, while trying to control the riot, supplied an escort to get the team to the bus. The windows were shattered, and everyone had to lie down on the floor.

We were faced with another huge problem, the team was expected to return for another game against South Vietnam the next night. Back in the hotel a meeting was held and the players voted to return home immediately. Who could have blamed them. The Australian Embassy insisted that it would be better if we played. No, was the players' firm reply to the diplomats.

In the middle of this impasse Peter stood up and made an impassioned speech, saying the decision was wrong and that the players owed it to themselves and to Australia to go out and play, not to be intimidated and show everyone the true spirit and guts of the Australian people. It was great stuff from Peter! And the result? The team returned the next day, won the game 1–0 and won over the crowd.

In 1978, the German Rudi Gutendorf assumed the mantle of Australian coach. I went to meet him and welcome him to Australia. His first comment to me was he believed we had a Dutch physio and I must get rid of him. I told him I wouldn't do it especially as he was a friend and had done nothing wrong. Gutendorf just glared.

His first training run with the Australian squad was in a camp about 30 kilometres out of town. As the practice started he turned to Peter and demanded to know why there weren't training bibs for the players to wear. Peter explained he didn't have any bibs because he hadn't been told to pack them. Gutendorf was furious and told him he wanted them immediately. I got the giggles as I thought of the prospect of getting in a car, travelling all the way back into town, trying to find bibs, then bringing them back — Peter would arrive back about four hours after training was finished. It gave Gutendorf an excuse to sack Peter, which he did.

We had a team reunion a few years ago and Peter turned up as cantankerous and impatient as ever. He died from cancer in 2003; I miss him a lot.

'Frank Arok was an inveterate showman who couldn't help himself if a newspaper photographer was around.'

27. THE GOOD, THE BAD AND THE MAD

THERE HAVE BEEN 14 coaches of the Socceroos since I first started as the doctor for the Australian team in 1967. Of these, some were very good, several were fine, one was considered hopeless, some people reckoned one was a conman and others thought one was a bit barmy.

The problem is that whenever you make a list of the best this or the best that, people will immediately say someone either should or should not be on it. To a large extent, any such list is a personal and subjective one, making it biased, uninformed, even stupid, if you like, but it's yours. And for those who don't like it — well, make up your own list.

A few years ago, the venerable London *Times* magazine published its list of the 100 best cricketers of all time and Sir Donald Bradman was not only graded second, but he was also the only Australian in the first twelve. Fourth on the list was Alfred Mynn. Don't feel too bad if you have never heard of him, he was born in England in 1807 and was supposed to have invented over-arm bowling. I'm told he would offer the advice 'Beef and beer are the things to play cricket on'. The so-called expert list was compiled by an Englishman.

The other important point is that no Test batsman has an average of 100 per cent. Even the great Bradman missed out on that score. So there have to be good points and bad points, as an Australian soccer president once said to a coach, 'We probably will keep you on while your good points continue to be greater than your bad ones.' You can concentrate on any coach's bad points and say he was no good; or you can concentrate on his good points and say how effective you think he is, or rather was. You pay your money and you take your choice. I have no intention of trying to convince anybody about my choices.

The coach has to tread many different and difficult paths. It is not only a case of technical knowledge, expertise or experience. He has to face many other different problems: political, interstate rivalry, rumours, lies, innuendo, jealousy. On top of all that, someone may not like the way he speaks or dresses. He has to succeed with one eye kept firmly on his back. It is also imperative that he has a heavy — a top soccer politician — as his minder and mentor, as Rale Rasic found out when he lost his. Above all the most needed quality of all would be luck, good luck.

If, in the unlikely eventuality I was ever elected to the position of soccer supremo, the first thing I would order would be to ban all coaches from screaming and shouting instructions from the sidelines at the players on the field. I've heard them do it thousands of times, but know of only two occasions when it resulted in any significant difference. The coaches are really doing it for their own benefit, not for the players, who often cannot even understand them among all the background noise. Worse still, I have often seen a player about to kick a ball when the shout comes from the bench to do something different and he falls between both options and ends up doing neither. The player then cops the blame. After all, player and coach are both looking at the circumstances from a different perspective, seeing opponents from different angles.

Nearly all of the coaches do it, and Frank Arok was as bad as any. One day he was shouting at the players, who were becoming visibly more upset about it. They came off at half-time, seething and threatening serious revolt. The players, led by David Ratcliffe, marched straight up to Frank and started off belligerently, 'Listen, Frank, we can't keep playing with all your shouting.'

'You listen son, you are paid to play and I am paid to shout. So you get on with your playing and I'll get on with my shouting.'

Even David had to laugh, and the situation was defused, if not resolved.

I will have to leave Frank Farina out of my list of the best coaches for a few reasons. I've not worked with him as coach, and he is still at the very beginning of his career. I feel there is an extremely good chance, given adequate funding and support, he will turn out to be not only one of our very best coaches, but a local one too. It is well past the time we abandoned our cultural cringe that insists upon importing foreign coaches.

I have already written at some length about Rale Rasic, the only coach ever to get us to the World Cup and the much under-rated Joe Vlasits. Dr Joe Venglos should also be mentioned before I head to my first choice.

JOE VENGLOS WOULD probably be top of the list, except he was only in Australia for one series, three games against Scotland in 1967. He had a great deal going for him. He was young — so he could relate well with the players — intelligent, and had played for his native Bratislava and Czechoslovakia.

He lived in Australia for some three years as coach of Prague club in the Sydney competition, so he also knew the local scene. He was driven out because our draconian system refused to recognise his impressive experience and European university qualifications in Physical Education, forcing him to work in a factory. He had dearly wanted to stay and told me he and his wife would have loved to have lived in Australia and bring the kids up here, but it was not to be. He returned to his native Czechoslovakia, became their national coach, won the European Championship and took the team to the World Cup. He did come back here on a lecture tour for FIFA in 1977, and I accompanied him for some of it, but he couldn't talk about his life because a Czech secret service man accompanied him everywhere he went.

Later Joe hoped to get the coaching job here after Frank Arok left in 1990. It also seemed he was not too worried about how much money would be offered, but the soccer politicians blocked that move and he was lost to Australian Soccer.

Intriguingly, one of the first things Frank Lowy did when he assumed the leadership of Australian Soccer in 2003 was to invite Venglos back in 2004 to lay down a blueprint for the work confronting the country's new technical director. It was perhaps predictable that a man with Lowy's unabashed love of the game, and unashamed love of his adopted country, Australia, should turn to Venglos.

This brings us to Frank Arok, coach from 1983 to 1989. I was looking for just a couple of words to describe him, but find it impossible. Arok was dedicated, intelligent, plain-speaking and controversial. More than any other coach I have ever met he was prepared to let the players take the glory when they won and he would take the blame when they lost.

Frank Arok was also an inveterate showman who couldn't help himself if a newspaper photographer was around. This could be misinterpreted as self-promotion, but he almost always used it to promote his Socceroos. Many people disliked Frank and his style, although that never seemed to worry him too much. He was happily married and liked nothing better than to be at home with his lovely wife, Gordana.

Whenever our team played away, Frank would relax on the last day by finding a casino and he always demanded that someone accompany him. I had that dubious honour a few times, but usually was able to dodge it, because I hate gambling and, to me, casinos are the most boring places in the world. He always played roulette and, by my standards, would often bet heavily. Although I didn't know much about it, I could see that he was not much of a player, often gambling recklessly, but he enjoyed it and it seemed to distract him from re-living the game that had just been played.

Frank was a physical education teacher in Yugoslavia where he played football. When an injury finished that career, he began coaching at the age of 27 and within two years was the coach of the first division club Novi Sad, at the same time he worked as a sports journalist. In 1968, he came to Sydney's St George Budapest club for the first of his stints of coaching. In 1983 Les Scheinflug was coach of the Australian senior and youth teams, and the youth team was away playing in the Youth World Cup in Mexico. This left a gap for a senior coach for the team in Australia to play that year against England and the game's administrators, led by Sir Arthur George who was no fan of Scheinflug, chose Arok to fill it. Arok showed his masterful tactical skill, sorting out where England liked to attack and how to block them. Time and again I have seen him plan seemingly minor changes in attack or defence to make a huge difference to a result. And so it happened against England, resulting in scores of 0–0, 0–1 and 1–1 — tremendous results for a series in which England had expected a whitewash.

Thus began a great era for the Socceroos highlighted by wins against Argentina, Yugoslavia, Israel, New Zealand and South Korea. Arok's

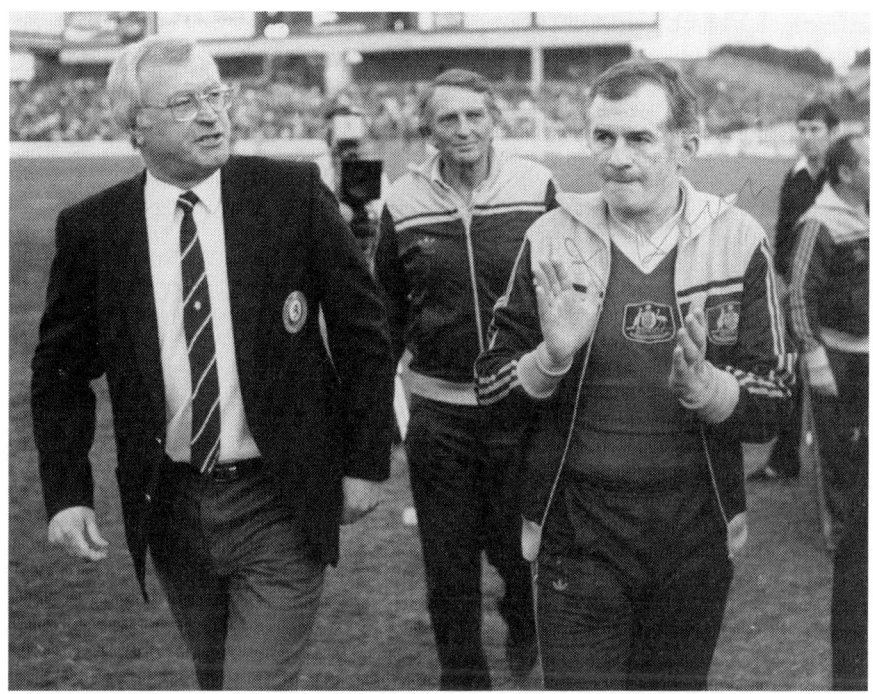

Leaving Melbourne Olympic Park with Frank Arok after he engineered a brilliant tactical draw against England, 1983. (BRIAN CORRIGAN'S COLLECTION)

victories were a result of meticulous planning, knowledge of the opposition and the psychology required to out-think them.

In 1985 the Socceroos played against Israel, who in the past had always provided bitter encounters. On the way to Israel, the team stopped off in Athens where they were invited to attend a game between Greece and Italy. I was sitting next to an Italian who kept telling me that Italy had no hope, because he knew the Greeks had bribed the referee. When Greece scored the first goal, he said he had told me so. However the Italians ended up winning 2–1 and when I turned to ask him what he thought of that he had disappeared. Maybe he was lucky, for outside a riot had begun. We were finally given an escort and told we must all stick together. When we arrived back at the bus, Frank was missing. Some time later, Frank turned up at the hotel, having pushed his way though a throng of angry Greeks. Riot. What riot? It seemed that Frank did not have a care in the world.

The mind games began when we arrived in Israel and Frank played his masterpiece, a dummy, as he loved to call it. At the last practice on the day before the match the players were told that places in the team for the game had not been settled, they were up for grabs and Frank suggested it would all depend on the vigour they showed during the final practice session. They did not need to be told twice and went in boots and all. It was horrific and I had visions of being up all night treating the smashed limbs. The Israeli scouts and newspapermen stood with their mouths agape, asking, 'Do you always train like this?'

'Oh, no,' said Frank, straight-faced. 'I decided to give them a light run before the game. It's usually much rougher than this.'

They were shattered, and their newspapers next morning predicted an Israeli bloodbath. The Australian team went out next day and played good constructive football, while the Israelis ran all around the park trying to kill them.

The second dummy Frank played was at a pre-match news conference where Frank suddenly announced that Eddie Krncevic, the Australian striker who was playing in Belgium, would be joining the squad. Of course, Frank had no means of getting Krncevic from Belgium to play in the game, but his comment caused a great deal of consternation for the Israeli coach. The Israelis had one of their best teams ever and did not want any of their plans to be altered.

Frank placed me in a difficult position on the day of the game. Not long before lunch he told me to go and check the kitchen to see if the team was going to be poisoned. I burst out laughing. I was convinced he was playing one of his famous dummies. That really upset Frank and I quickly realised he was deadly serious when he ordered me, in no uncertain terms, to do what I had been told. Now, one of the very first things I always did when the team arrived at any strange or new place was to look at the kitchen and get to know the chef, it usually paid dividends. This chef had been particularly helpful in arranging any small thing a player preferred and I didn't like to go now and insult him by telling him I was there to check on whether or not he was poisoning us. I knew there were many stories floating around about such deliberate skullduggery, but I could not imagine this guy allowing such a trick. What to do? I went to him and explained my problem. He laughed, just as I had, showed me the smorgasbord and pasta dish he had prepared and asked, 'Do you want to taste it?' I just shook my head and told him I'd take his word for it. Of course, I told Frank I had tasted it, and, sure enough, no one became ill after lunch.

It was, predictably, a very tough game with the Israelis taking more dives than a surfer at Bondi. Two Australians were dismissed. One was Ken Murphy with a red card, the other Frank Arok, although for a rather strange reason. An Israeli player went over the ball, crunching into Steve O'Connor's shin. The referee awarded a free kick to the Israelis and followed that up by giving Steve the yellow card. Frank was on his feet protesting, justifiably, the incredible decision. The referee was not interested and, determined to put his stamp on the game, aggressively waved Frank away. The referee may or may not have understood English, but Frank most certainly thought he didn't and shouted: '[Expletive deleted] you' and a few more unprintable words. Big mistake! He was immediately sent from the field. The ref may not have understood English, but he certainly understood body language. I walked with Frank to where we had to stand and watch the game from behind a barbed wire fence in the company of hundreds of fist-waving, screaming Israelis. The goalkeeper, Terry Greedy, also had to come off with an horrific gash above his left eye which was the result of an accidental Australian boot.

After all that, Australia won the game 2–1.

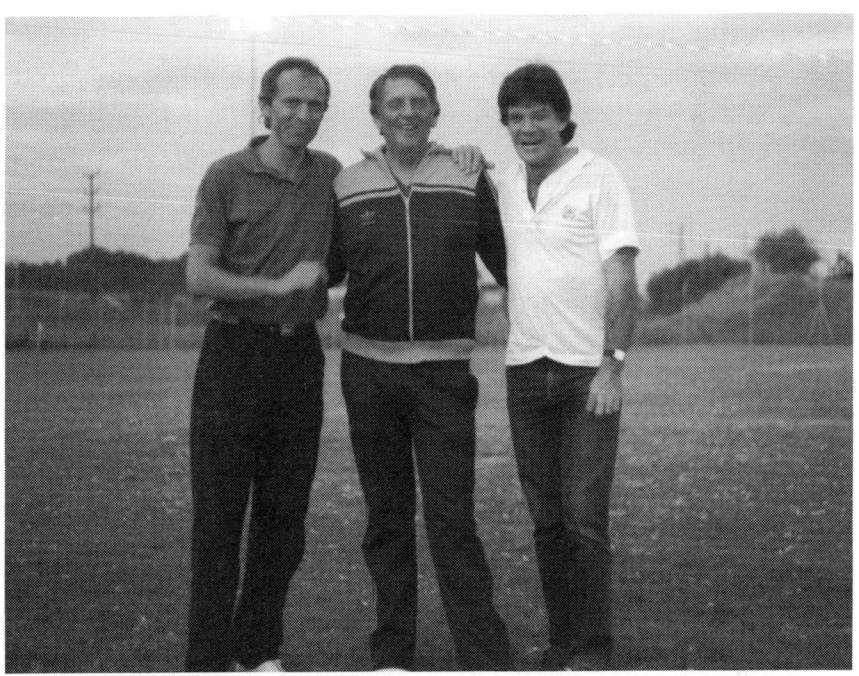

In Israel in 1985 catching up with two great ex-captains, Israel's Mordechai Spiegler (left) and Australia's John Warren (right). (BRIAN CORRIGAN COLLECTION)

THERE WAS A news conference after we arrived back in Sydney which also caused Frank some angst. During it, he used one of his favourite expressions 'mad dog' and the news agencies quickly flashed the term around the world. Ironically, on this occasion, Frank was using the expression to describe himself. At the end of 1985, we were playing Scotland for a World Cup berth. The first match was in Glasgow and the British media turned up in droves. It was one of the biggest attendances for a news conference and not just football writers, but a large contingent of Fleet Street journalists, all set to crucify the 'mad dog'. Frank, being a trained journalist, turned everything around with his discussion on tactics. In the end he had them all eating out of his hand and saying what a fine, intelligent coach we had. It was beautiful to watch.

The World Cup qualifying game, played on a bitterly cold Glaswegian night at Hampden Park, ended with the Socceroos losing 2–0. We have heard talk in recent years about the Australian cricket team being a bunch of sledgers, but they are amateurs compared with the fans on the terraces during that game. The Scottish crowd, although basically good-natured, were expert sledgers who set about trying to upset the Australians, but the Socceroos loved the atmosphere and found the fans' songs vastly amusing. The most popular ditty was 'You're just a bunch of [pause] sheep shaggers'. They were confusing us with the Kiwis, surely. Mostly the songs were to do with our convict origins, how none of us had ever known our father and what the Scots in Australia were doing to our wives. I couldn't understand many of the songs because they were sung in the broad Glaswegian vernacular. Some were so ribald that I would not dare repeat them here, such as what they would do to Matilda, sung to strains of our national 'anthem' 'Waltzing Matilda'.

ON THE PLANE trip home, Frank was plotting the return match in Australia.

'We'll play it in Darwin or Cairns,' he decided. 'And on a very bumpy pitch. They won't be able to play their style of game under those conditions. And the heat and humidity will kill them. They would do exactly the same if the circumstances were reversed.'

Frank's suggestion fell on deaf ears. Could you believe it? The soccer hierarchy wasn't interested in the final result, even if a spot in the World Cup finals was up for grabs, which would have netted us millions of dollars. No, it was played at night in Melbourne. Frank was livid and demanded to know why.

'Well, after all, it's Melbourne's turn to have a game,' was the official answer.

To use one of Frank's favourite expressions: Unbelievable! It could only happen with soccer in Australia. No stinking hot and humid tropical weather. No bumpy pitch. We managed a nil–all draw. Another World Cup campaign down the drain.

THE BICENTENNIAL YEAR, 1988, placed a tremendous load on the Socceroos. Frank quickly realised what a difficult time lay ahead, having to play quality opposition while having to peak some five times during the year. So he devised a horror course, a commando course he called it, which was a huge fitness program twice a day, six days a week for a month. The players grumbled and almost buckled at the knees, but they completed it. Later in the year they realised the sense of it all.

During that year the Socceroos went to Seoul for the Olympics. There has never been a prouder man in all Australia than Frank Arok, he almost burst with pride. Time and time again he told the players what a great honour it was for them to be going to represent Australia.

There was a big reception for all the Olympians just before we flew out for Seoul and Frank, for the first time that I ever saw it happen, had a few drinks. He certainly didn't drink a lot that night, but he was very relaxed and merry, as were members of his team, as we boarded the plane. This did not go down at all well with the other highly disciplined Olympic athletes, who disdainfully looked down on the Socceroos as clowns. This was sad because they were really doing no harm and they had never previously been allowed to drink on a plane. I think it was mostly to do with Frank being so happy just to be part of an Olympic team.

It took a lot of time and hard work in the Village and on the pitch to recover the lost respect. In the qualifying matches they beat Yugoslavia 1–0, then lost 3–0 to the eventual silver medallists Brazil, before beating Nigeria 1–0. The Socceroos were eventually knocked out in the quarter-finals, beaten 3–0 by the Soviet Union, who went on to win gold. The Aussies were placed fifth. After that the team could have treated the rest of the Olympics as a holiday. Instead they formed cheer squads to go and barrack for other Australian teams still competing. This went a very long way towards rebuilding respect in the eyes of the other Olympians.

IN 1989 FRANK fell foul of the soccer politicians. He had certainly given them some excuses over the years and he had not been successful in seeking out the Holy Grail of Australian soccer — qualifying for the World Cup finals. The ASF told him he had to apply for his own job, knowing that he was a very proud man who would never contemplate doing this. And he didn't. He'd had many previous coaching jobs without ever having to apply for them. He had never signed a contract, preferring a gentleman's agreement, for his word was his bond and he would not deign to argue over money. After his last game, a 3–0 victory over Moscow Torpedo in Melbourne on 2 February 1990, the players and support staff pitched in for a beautiful, suitably inscribed gift, presented during an emotional farewell in the dressing-room. From the ASF there was nothing.

Frank Arok was a master tactician, a planner, a long way ahead of and able to out-think rival coaches, a good motivator, and bubbling with various ideas. Australian soccer owed him a huge debt of gratitude for under him it had come of age, mainly as a result of the self-belief and confidence he had instilled in his players.

He had so much more to give, but he was gone.

'He said he had to get the heart of a dead animal ... and on the night of a full moon, he had to drive a stake through it. He would then be cured.'

28. MY FRIEND, THE WITCH DOCTOR

THE MIND IS a powerful instrument that should never be underestimated as a cause or a cure of illness. Three times I have been involved in a problem associated with witch doctors to demonstrate the truth of this statement.

At one time, I travelled around the Northern Territory with my great school friend, John Cumming, who had become a legend in Alice Springs. Some of the old locals I met in a bar spoke about him with awe, explaining how he had worked as a fettler on the railway for £5 a week before coming into the Alice and starting a chemist shop in the days when the Territory used to prohibit such private enterprise (even though John had a pharmacy degree). He also took to prospecting, made a lot of money and became very friendly with some local Aboriginal people, so much so that they made him one of their blood brothers.

One day, far from Alice Springs, John and I went to visit them and they said they would put on a corroboree in a dry creek bed that evening in our honour. One chap was sitting in a corner, his head in his hands, saying absolutely nothing to anyone. He looked terribly ill, very thin and wasted and I asked what had happened to him and could I help? They said he was going to die and no treatment at all could help him.

'Why, what is wrong?'

It turned out that he was from a nearby tribe and had become involved with the wife of someone important in that group, breaking one of their strict Aboriginal laws. He had been forced to flee to avoid being killed and was now hiding out here, but an elder — they used a name like *kadicha* — had pointed the bone at him to cast a spell. Members of the tribe were now singing him to death from far away.

'How can they do that?'

The people I was with said his head had been lifted up and turned around the other way. Nothing could be done for him now, he would just fade away and die some time the next day. And he did!

WHEN WORKING IN England in 1963, I was asked to see a promising young football player who had been invited to become an apprentice with a major English soccer team, much to the delight of his parents. There was a bit of a problem, however. He complained of a foot injury which prevented him from playing. He'd had many tests and treatments, none of which had made any difference. When I first saw him, I honestly could not find anything that appeared to be wrong with him and I was puzzled. He had some fairly non-specific treatment and I assured him and his parents that he should be showing some improvement in a month or so.

When I saw him after a month he announced, not too unhappily I thought, that he was much worse and could barely walk and certainly could not play football. Again, I could not detect any evidence of damage. I asked the parents to leave the room, looked him straight in the eye and said there was nothing wrong with his foot and he should tell me what had been happening to him. With this, he burst out crying and with tears running down his face said, 'If I tell you, you must promise not to tell my parents.'

'Most definitely,' I replied.

The story he told was that the other apprentices hated him because he was an outsider and wanted him out of the squad as his presence meant that one of their friends could not be included. They did not see why their mate's only chance of making a life for himself should be ruined by an intruder. Most of these players were descendants of Caribbean families and they had consulted a witch doctor and took great delight in telling our young hero that he would have a foot injury that would prevent him from playing.

MY FRIEND, THE WITCH DOCTOR | 197

'Do you know what can be done to overcome this spell?' I asked him.

He smiled for the first time and said that he had found out the correct method. He said he had to get the heart of a dead animal, which he could obtain easily as his father was a butcher, and at a crossroad on the night of a full moon, he had to drive a stake through it. He would then be cured. I had to admit I had never heard of such a remedy before and thought it would never work.

Next time I saw him, he walked in smiling. He told me he had carried out these instructions and his foot was better, but he was not going to return to that squad. As it turned out, he never did. Soon afterwards, he was involved in a car accident, broke a leg and never played again. Read into that whatever you will.

THE THIRD INCIDENT occurred in 1969 in Lorenco Marques (now Maputo) the capital of Mozambique when that country was still under Portuguese rule. The Socceroos were there to play two matches against Rhodesia, as it was then known before it became Zimbabwe. We thought we would have an easy victory and be able to fly to Israel to playoff for a place in the 1970 World Cup. At the time there was a ban on anybody playing in Rhodesia for political reasons, so we had to play the matches in neighbouring Mozambique.

After Australia had played both matches, we were faced with a major problem. Both were drawn, 1–1 and 0–0. Not only were the Rhodesians seemingly allowed to kick us to death, but also they had a tall, gangly, uncoordinated goalkeeper named Jordan, who was either so brilliant or, much more likely, so hopeless that he kept falling over. Every time he did so, he would somehow manage to block one of our shots at goal, often with his feet.

Our problem was compounded because our management had assumed we would be flying out of there as soon as we had won the second game. And they were so confident that they had not bothered to book any alternative flights for us. The bottom line was that we had to win the third game to have any chance of reaching Israel in time for the deciding playoff. Our liaison officer, a man with the felicitous name of Fernando Fernandes, came to the rescue. He was the local representative for United Press International (UPI), and had his office in the most opulent bordello in all Lorenco Marques.

It was an establishment well known on the African continent. Every Friday night, two Boeing 707 planes full of white South African men would arrive to spend the entire weekend with the black ladies employed there. I happened to mention this when we arrived back in South Africa en route to Israel, but nobody believed me. Some people there wanted me whipped for telling such ridiculous lies about their menfolk, who would never even think of doing such a thing. They frowned when I suggested they go there to see for themselves.

Anyway, Fernando offered to find the local witch doctor who would help our cause. It was arranged that I would meet this man at the football stadium at dawn, never my best time, the following morning.

Right at dawn, Fernando and I were standing in the appointed place behind the goalposts. Suddenly, without our having seen or heard his approach, our man was standing beside us. It was the most eerie feeling. I had felt certain he would be dressed in the exotic tribal garb witch doctors always wear in the movies. Instead he was immaculately dressed in a Savile Row suit. I felt quite disappointed.

'Good morning, sir,' he said in a beautiful Oxford accent. 'I already know your problem and I can fix it.' I was most impressed with that for an opener.

'How will you do that?'

'Well, I just plant this bag of bones behind the goalpost pointing straight at the goalkeeper's heart.' I looked at him quizzically, but he didn't bat an eyelid. 'If you are thinking that he has to change ends at half-time, I can tell you now it will make no difference.'

'OK,' I nodded. 'We'll go back to the hotel and Fernando here will arrange to put it into the newspapers, so the black players in the Rhodesian team will find out what we have done.'

My newfound black medical partner turned a deadly shade of grey, 'Oh, no, you can't do that, Sir. The Portuguese would cut off my hand.'

I had to agree, but reluctantly because the whole idea had been to make sure the story was in the newspapers.

'That will be £50 Sterling, please, Sir.'

It was now me who turned a whiter shade of pale.

'The team manager handles all those matters. You'll have to see him about that,' I explained, knowing that the sum of money was about all the spare cash the team had. Our teams really did work on the proverbial shoestring budget in those days.

We raced back to the hotel where the Rhodesian team were having breakfast. I made sure they knew where we had been and what had been done on our behalf by the witch doctor. I can't say for certain whether it worked or not, but they did seem mightily impressed. And we did win the decider easily 3–1 with their goalie having a very ordinary game.

We still had a problem, as we still had to get to Johannesburg to catch our flight to Israel, and the next commercial flight from Mozambique would not be for a couple of days. Alternative transport had to be arranged. When we arrived at the airport at dawn the next morning, after a very long night celebrating, our hearts sank. Our transport was a tiny, one-engine plane. We could barely squeeze into it.

'That will never get us up over the mountains,' observed one astute traveller.

Suddenly the witch doctor appeared, standing beside the manager asking for his money, but the manager, who had probably had a rougher night than anyone else, refused to talk to him.

'You will be sorry, Sir, because I can put a spell on this plane.'

'Pay him his money,' the players were all yelling, but the manager remained completely unmoved. Right at that moment there was a flash of lightning that lit up the airport. You have never in your life seen so many terrified footballers (and team doctor) and we didn't relax until we finally landed in Johannesburg. To this day, the then Australian captain, Johnny Warren believes that the spell cast that morning still haunts Australian soccer.

You don't believe it? Well, what other explanation can there be for the perennial troubles that have inflicted it ever since, preventing its development?

'A horse trampled his big toe ... it was squashed flat as a tack, broken in several places, the toenail was pulled off ... "Don't worry about it, Doc, just put a Band-Aid on it".'

29. BLOOD AND GUTS

HEROIC DEEDS ARE often the stuff of history books. Courage on the battlefield or during national emergencies such as bushfires is well recognised as a supremely selfless act carried out without, or more accurately despite, fear. It may be rewarded with a Victoria Cross or some other medal or award, or just remembered by the hero's mates. Initiation rites to transform a boy into a man may demand some feat of heroism, such as boys from the Masai tribe having to find and kill a lion.

Courage is also well recognised on the sports field, where it is usually referred to as guts. Sport requires many other attributes besides talent, including dedication, the will to win, fitness and luck — to mention a few — but as important as any of these would be guts. How do you define guts and a gutsy performance? It may remain difficult to define, but when it happens it is immediately recognised by everyone who witnesses it and usually involves having to play on through fear or pain without self-aggrandisement.

Guts differs from toughness, for there are plenty of tough but not particularly brave characters out there on the sport field on any given day. The axiom that adorns many a dressing-room wall, and is so beloved by coaches states that 'when the going gets tough, the tough get going'. There are some tough people who quickly turn it in when the going gets really tough. There is one such character who would be on most people's list of tough guys. I saw him hit a lot of people, but never, ever anyone bigger than himself. No names, no pack drill.

Many qualify for the title of being the toughest I have ever seen play. My list would always include John Sattler, the front-row enforcer from South Sydney. There is the story of him playing against Manly in the 1970 Rugby League grand final, when he was captain of the Rabbitohs. Just 4 minutes into game, Sattler was king-hit by John Bucknell, and his jaw was broken in several places. Somehow the punch went unnoticed by the referee. Sattler didn't leave the field, but played on with his drooping, bloodied jaw for the rest of the game, still doing his full share of tackling (and not afraid to being tackled himself). Others have played on with broken bones, but considering all the circumstances, this was one of the gutsiest performances I have ever seen.

Gutsiness also differs from foolhardiness, an action that might appeal to the crowd as being tough, but one where the odds are surely just not worth it. There are two examples of that, both involving Rugby League fullbacks. One was the great Clive Churchill who, one day at Redfern Oval, was knocked unconscious and had to be carried from the field. It was in the days when replacements weren't allowed. After about half an hour he appeared running, no, that's not the word, tottering down the stairs. The crowd cheered, went wild.

'Surely they can't let him go back on,' I said to one of the Souths officials who did not understand what I was talking about. The result was inevitable, no brownie points were awarded out there for a courageous but obviously foolhardy act. The first time Churchill handled the ball, whack, and he was carried off unconscious again. This time he couldn't return. Gutsy or foolhardy?

Bob Batty, a Manly fullback, wouldn't have weighed 70 kilograms when he stepped out of a shower. One day he hit one of the huge Balmain front-row forwards, not really a clever idea. Balmain was given a free kick just as the fulltime bell sounded. The ball was put high in the air, Bob was under it and two massive Balmain forwards went right over the top of him. I thought he could have dodged the ball, after all the game was over. He stood his ground. He couldn't walk for a month. Gutsy or foolhardy?

Sometimes the dividing line can become blurred. The first Olympic women's marathon was run in Los Angeles in 1984. Who could ever forget the sight of the American-based Swiss runner, Gabriele Andersen-Scheiss, after she entered the stadium and for the next 5 or 6 minutes staggered and stumbled all over the track? Everyone agonised about what to do. Officials were not allowed to go to her aid because that would mean instant disqualification. Her doctor in the stand was refused permission to get onto the track. He told me later that he would have stopped her determined attempt to reach the finishing line at all costs as he feared she was having a stroke. Many who witnessed it agreed that was likely to happen. She finally collapsed over the line. The rules were subsequently altered to allow medical help in such circumstances. She did recover, but never ran again. Gutsy or foolhardy?

NONETHELESS THERE ARE so many clear-cut examples of gutsy performances on the sporting field it is difficult to know where to begin.

In cricket, we have the sight of Rick McCosker coming in to bat when his team needed him in the Centenary Test against England in Melbourne in 1977, his swollen face was bound up in a bandage after Bob Willis had earlier broken his jaw.

Or Bobby Simpson coming back at the age of 41 to captain Australia when they had to go to the West Indies in 1978 to face their awesome speed bowlers.

Or Colin Cowdrey making a comeback in 1974 because the English team was in such trouble against Dennis Lillee and Jeff Thomson, facing the short-pitched deliveries as well as any of his team-mates, despite the body blows he received. Cowdrey was a few days short of his 42nd birthday and had not played a Test for more than three years. Four days after arriving in Australia he had to face the two fast bowlers on their favourite Perth pitch.

The Olympics can usually be relied on to produce a host of gutsy performances, such as the heroics of the New Zealand hockey keeper, Trevor Manning at Montreal, playing with a shattered kneecap. Another example, from the same Olympics in 1976, was the Japanese gymnastics gold medal winner, Shun Fujimoto, who fractured his right knee while performing the floor routine in the team event. Despite the intense pain the 26-year-old told neither his team-mates nor his coach. He realised that he needed to keep going as the top five scores from the six-man team counted, and he didn't want to leave his team short. He moved on to the pommel horse on which he scored a 9.5, then came the rings. This required real guts, as his routine called for a twisting, triple somersault dismount at great speed. As he did the dismount he tore ligaments and completely dislocated the knee to add to the fracture. Only then did his team realise something was amiss. He still scored a personal best 9.7 on the rings. The Japanese beat the Soviet Union by 576.85 to 576.45 to win gold. Interviewed some years later Fujimoto was asked if he would go through such pain again for a medal. His answer was a simple, 'No way.'

BILL ROYCROFT WAS 45 when he won an equestrian gold medal at the 1960 Rome Olympics. He really was a typical laconic Australian bushman, tougher than the day is long. When his horse, Our Solo, fell during the cross-country discipline of the three-day event, Bill suffered concussion and a broken right collarbone and had to be admitted to hospital. The following day, defying doctors' orders, Roycroft rode in the final section, the show-jumping. Had he not done so, Australia, down to just two other riders could not have taken advantage of their good position to win the teams' event. Roycroft had to be lifted into the saddle. He had no use of his right arm and was in agony as his horse took each hurdle. He never showed his pain and rode a faultless round over the 12 obstacles, helping pave the way for a gold medal for himself and team-mates Laurie Morgan and Neale Lavis.

Roycroft also competed with his son Wayne in 1968 and 1976, taking the bronze medal on each occasion. He was at Munich in 1972 with another son, Clarke, when the Australians finished fourth. As a tribute to this outstanding family, Old Bill, as he was known, was accorded the rare honour of carrying the Australian flag for the Opening Ceremony in the 1968 Mexico Olympics. In the morning, not long before we were to leave for the march, a horse trampled his big toe. You can imagine the mess a horse can make of a human toe. It was squashed flat as a tack and broken in several places. The toenail was pulled off and blood was oozing out.

'Bill, how on earth are you going to march with that, let alone carry the flag?' I asked.

'Don't worry about it, Doc, just put a Band-Aid on it.' A Band-Aid? It was dressed as well as possible considering his swollen foot had to be squeezed into a shoe.

'No pain-killers thanks, Doc. Might make me a bit drowsy.'

So he marched carrying the heavy Australian flag. A simple thing like a big toe smashed all over the place was not going to stop him. Proud, upright, never once letting on to anyone, never limping, he must have been in awful agony. Gutsy? You bet!

ABEBE BIKILA WAS an Ethiopian marathon runner who competed in three Olympics. At the first in Rome in 1960, he was a virtually unknown 28-year-old, having run only three marathons in his life. For trivia buffs, it was intriguing that he was born on 7 August 1932, the day the marathon was run at the first Los Angeles Olympics. Bikila ran barefoot just weeks after having his appendix out, and in the heat of a Rome evening won in a then world's best time of 2 hours 15 minutes 16.2 seconds. He then sat down in the middle of the Olympic stadium and performed a series of exercises! It was also the first Olympic marathon to be won by an African. It was said Abebe got his inspiration about 1500 metres from home by seeing the obelisk of Axum, which had been plundered from Ethiopia by Fascist Italy in 1937.

In Tokyo four years later, the Ethiopians managed to find Bikila a pair of sandshoes and socks and again he ran a world's best, this time 2 hours 12 minutes 11.2 seconds. It seemed he had won effortlessly as he finished more than 4 minutes faster than the silver medal winner, Basil Heatley of Great Britain. Employed as a member of the Ethiopian Imperial Household Guard for his beloved Emperor Haile Selassie, Bikila came to Mexico as the race favourite in 1968. Australia's then world-record marathon runner, Derek Clayton, had no realistic chance of winning at altitude.

I used to spend some time in Mexico City with a Mexican stand-by X-ray technician. He told me that he was a bit bored as he was never busy. So I suggested that I would teach him English in return for him teaching me Spanish. The X-ray department worked on the well-known Mexican 'manana' principle, so it could take ages to get any results, but because of our friendship, he provided a very quick service for our team, which was a big help at times.

I was waiting for him in his office one day when I noticed an X-ray on his desk of Abebe Bikila's leg. Naturally enough, I took a look at it and saw a stress fracture just above the ankle. Knowing the system, I realised that it would not be reported on for days. I raced back to our headquarters, very

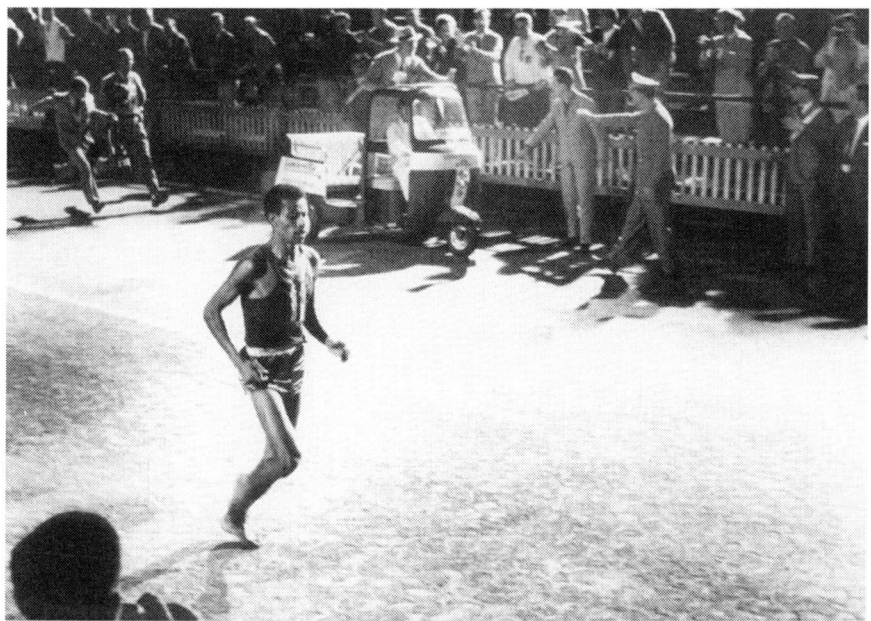

That extraordinary Olympian, Ethiopian marathon runner, Abeba Bikila, here winning gold at the 1960 Rome Olympics. He also won gold at Tokyo in 1964 but had to withdraw from the Mexico Olympic marathon (after running 17 kilometres!) because of a stress fracture above the ankle.
(AAP IMAGE/SPORT THE LIBRARY/PRESSE SPORTS)

satisfied that I was the only one at that stage to know that Bikila would not be able to compete. I told Derek Clayton, but he said he thought Abebe would still start the race. And he did, limping to the starting line, and running for 17 kilometres on his fracture before having to withdraw. When asked about his courageous performance trying to run in such obvious agony, Bikila replied simply, 'The public expect me to run.'

Bikila's life took a turn for the worse the following year. Driving a Volkswagen given to him by the emperor after his second gold medal, he crashed, broke his neck and severed his spinal cord, which left him a paraplegic confined to a wheelchair. Four years later he died of a brain haemorrhage. He was just 41 years of age.

OF THE THREE greatest examples of gutsy people I have personally encountered on the sporting field, Ron Clarke would be my top choice because he put his life on the line so valiantly.

The others on my list are David Hookes and Ken 'Slasher' Mackay.

Hookes broke into the Australian cricket team in 1977 for the Ashes Centenary Test, Australia against England at the Melbourne Cricket Ground, where he distinguished himself by hitting five fours in one over off the English captain, Tony Greig. Hookes was a fine batsman and when he retired had scored the highest number of Sheffield Shield runs (12,671) in the history of the famous competition. His Test appearances, 23, were limited as selectors felt his best batting was confined to the Adelaide Oval and, could you believe it, he did not bat *slowly* enough. Ironically, his batting style would have fitted in very well with the way the current Australian team play their cricket.

I was fortunate to see him playing against Victoria at the Adelaide Oval in 1982 when he scored a century in a record 43 minutes off only 34 balls. He had already scored a century (137) in the first innings; and South Australia was chasing 271 late on the last afternoon of the game. The Victorian fieldsmen were strung along the boundary, but he kept hitting fours and sixes between them. To no avail, he was dismissed for 107, with his team all out for 206. He told us later that every shot he played that day went exactly where he had wanted it to go.

JUST AFTER THE Centenary Test, World Series Cricket was set up and Hookes joined it along with the general exodus of Australian players. Was there ever a more aptly named cricketer? Hookes loved to play the hook shot, and the fierce, ruthless West Indian fast bowler Andy Roberts was only too happy to oblige by bowling short at him. Roberts could bowl two different types of bumpers — a very fast one but also a cleverly disguised slower one. Both types were aimed straight at the batsman's head. One particular day, while playing at the Sydney Showground, Roberts served up the slower one, and Hooksie went to hook it, but he was too early with his shot and the ball cannoned into his jaw. When I got out onto the ground to check him out, Hooksie was looking particularly unwell with a very swollen jaw and was trying to talk.

'I'm all right, just leave me alone,' he mumbled through gritted teeth.

'Spit,' I said. And he spat out a huge amount of blood and what looked like a bit of tooth. That finally convinced David to stop arguing and come off.

The ambulance on duty at the ground was nowhere to be found, so Mr Packer told us to get into his Jaguar and he would act as ambulance driver and take us to the hospital. No ambulance with blaring sirens could have been as fast as this, as the three of us drove up the wrong side of the road en route to St Vincent's Hospital. As we approached Oxford Street the traffic lights had just turned red, and as we were hurtling through the lights, Packer suddenly realised that we were heading into a one-way street ... the wrong way. He hit the brakes, they jammed, and the Jaguar stalled in the middle of Oxford Street. Panic stations. We managed to get the big bloke's Jaguar started and we made it to the hospital in one piece, well, sort of — one of us had a very broken jaw.

Hookes was unable to play for some time and with his jaw wired he lost a lot of weight, as he couldn't eat. When he eventually returned to play, it was, as though the Fates had so decreed, against the West Indies. He went out to bat and, of course, Andy Roberts was immediately brought on to bowl. Roberts' first ball was a bumper aimed straight at Hooksie's jaw. David hooked it straight over the fence for six, in a repeat of the shot he'd been attempting when he was injured. When the next ball was fired down the pitch, another bouncer headed for his jaw, it was also hooked over the fence, Andy called a truce. The performance that day took a lot of guts by David Hookes.

When his life was so cruelly, senselessly snuffed out in early 2004, the game lost one of its true free spirits.

ALL SPORTS HAVE their roll call of real life characters, but cricket always seems to have the most. Some time ago, I read an article written in the 1930s by the doyen of cricket writers, Neville Cardus, bemoaning the fact that there were no longer characters in the game like there had been in the 1910s and 1920s. I found this very strange and decided he must be wrong, until it dawned on me that he was reminiscing about teams he had been very closely associated with and had known the players really well. Of course, there are just as many characters in any era.

I was most involved with the teams in the 1960s and 1970s, so could write or tell more stories about players from that period. I am very sure there are just as many characters around out there now as there ever had been. Some are characters because they are great public entertainers. As a general rule, these players are also great characters in the privacy of the dressing-room, but let me assure you not all have the same personality off the field as they do on it. It also works the other way; some dour cricketers are very funny people off the field. Another problem can be those retired cricketers who are determined to prove that all top cricket finished the day after they retired and delight in denigrating today's players.

Ken Mackay is on my list of the greatest characters who ever played and also on my list of one of the gutsiest. Except to his family, he was never known by anything other than Slasher, the nickname given to him by team-mate, Aub Carrigan, when Mackay first played for Queensland. It was a satirical reference to how slowly Slasher could bat. Unloved by the media, he was always fully appreciated by his team-mates.

He had two special loves he was prepared to die for — one was his baggy green Australian cricket cap, the other his captain, Richie Benaud (you think that my hyperbole has gone too far, but my concern is that it may be an understatement). Mackay first played for Queensland as a bowler and batsman just after World War II, aged 21. He wasn't picked for the Australian team until 1956. He was noted for his defensive batting, but could bat much faster when required. In one match he played in Sydney there were four scores over 50, and his was the fastest. Yet the newspapers next day blasted him for scoring too slowly.

He certainly was easy to parody as he loped in carrying his heavy bat, chewing gum, with a bent-knee walk that reminded people of Groucho Marx or an American cowboy passing through the swing doors of a Wild West saloon. As he used to say, his job was to score runs, not look pretty and he certainly got that part right. His batting could best be described as distinctive — his knees flexed like a crab, heavy bat pointing straight ahead, ultra-short back lift ready to play defensively or to hit the loose ball with great timing, Slasher would appear to squirt the ball out like an orange pip. One secret to his success was that he was probably fitter than any one else going around at that time, allowing him to play on until he retired at the age of 37.

Slasher Mackey gets into my list for the occasion he probably would best be remembered for, an innings in Adelaide (more of that later), along with several other examples over a period of time.

When Richie Benaud became the Australian captain in 1958, he changed Slasher from a batsman (he had 6000 Shield runs for Queensland as a Number Three batsman) who bowled a bit into a bowling all-rounder.

In that role, as Richie says, 'He became a key man in the planning of my team.' Not many observers, even in the media, noted the significant change.

Throughout the entire 1956 Ashes tour, skipper Ian Johnson gave him only 132 overs to bowl, but on the 1959–60 tour to Pakistan and India, where two matches were played on the matting, he bowled brilliantly and his captain, Benaud, gave him almost as many as on that entire 1956 tour, with 123.4 overs, 169 runs for 10 wickets. In 1961, in the Oval Test alone he bowled 107 overs, taking seven wickets. On the whole tour, he tallied the most overs of any of Australia's bowlers, 667, 33 more than the next highest bowler, Alan Davidson, taking 52 wickets.

He also batted the least number of times, 25, of any of the recognised batsmen, and then often down the list between Davidson and Benaud. Except for playing against Middlesex at Lord's. In those days, the Lord's wicket had a notorious ridge running across in front of the batsman at the Nursery end. It worried the batsmen for it was right where a good length ball would land. An unplayable ball could turn up at any time. If the ball hit one side of the ridge, it leapt up at your throat. If it hit the other side, it shot along the ground. The really good bowlers, including Davidson, could exploit it unmercifully. Middlesex had one such good fast bowler, Alan Moss, who also played for England.

Nobody was in any hurry to open the innings that day.

'You open, Slash,' his skipper requested.

'OK, Rich,' Mackay replied, and buckled on his pads.

The first three batsmen to fall contributed a total of 15 runs between them as they found the ball whistling around their ears. The first ball from Moss to Slasher hit him on his knuckle, taking a large divot out of it.

'Shit!' said Slasher. But he wasn't going to stop batting just for that. This injury took a long time to heal.

'Don't tell Richie,' he said as I later helped tend to the wound.

Slasher's peculiar style suited the unusual situation perfectly. The rising ball he squirted away past point for four. The shooter always found his bat in the way. With 20 minutes to go until lunch, he was on 92 not out. This is absolutely perfect, I was thinking, I will make a fortune in the future betting that Slasher Mackay once made a century before lunch at Lord's. Everyone will take the bet because they will say that is impossible. Then he lost the strike to his great friend, Peter Burge, who struggled over those final 20 minutes up to lunch. Slasher saw little of the strike and did not score any more runs. He finished with 168 in four hours of batting, before falling to Moss.

The Marylebone Cricket Club (MCC) had always maintained the ridge was an illusion, or all part of a colonial plot to defame them, for they said that such a thing could never happen at Lord's. But it was there all right, and our players — and the English players — had the bruises all over their bodies to prove it.

After the Second Test at Lord's, a small army of MCC experts and surveyors examined the wicket with all their instruments and decided there was a ridge after all. There were then lots of theories as to why it was there. It was later shown to be due to subsidence from where a drainpipe ran and it could be fixed.

Another time, in 1958, Slasher was batting in Perth with Norm O'Neill against the MCC team. Norm was a great batsman, but a dreadful runner between wickets, especially if he was approaching his ton, as he was on this particular day. On 99 he called Slasher for a run. Slasher knew there was no run in it, but he sacrificed his own wicket rather than let Normie miss out on his hundred.

At Manchester in 1961, Australia retained the Ashes with a team that the English media had described — quite wrongly, as they found out to their acute embarrassment — as the worst ever to leave Australia. Australia was well behind in runs in the second innings and Benaud's strategy relied on containing their batsmen. Slasher bowled something like 14 consecutive overs for as many runs. At one stage, he was furious with himself because he had bowled a half-volley. Maybe that doesn't sound anything out of the box. But somewhere along the way Slasher tore a calf muscle. He ignored it and kept bowling. First over after tea, he took the prize wicket of Ken Barrington, and was given a spell at leg slip so he would not have to chase too many runs. One ball was heading for four, but Slasher took after it, painful leg and all, to cut it down to a three. Nobody out there would have blamed him for just jogging after it, but that wasn't Slasher's way of playing cricket.

His gutsiest effort was against the West Indies in Adelaide in 1961. At tea on the last day, the West Indians had the Test all but won with the Australian team down to the tail and struggling. Two quick wickets saw a Windies' victory being inevitable. This was the case as the last batsman with Slasher was to be Lindsay 'Spinner' Kline, a noted rabbit. He'd been out on the practice pitch trying to get his eye in, but called a halt to the session when he could hardly lay bat on ball.

Nevertheless, the two of them did survive until the final over, which was to be bowled by the Windies' fastest bowler, big Wes Hall coming back from a rest. That over lasted ten balls. There was the normal eight of that era, plus two no balls. Slasher had kept the strike. Facing the last ball, he withdrew his bat so he couldn't get a snick, stood up to Wes, and was hit a sickening thump above his heart. That effort of literally putting his body on the line is now part of Australian cricket folklore. And Slasher won the everlasting respect of his team-mates for such a gutsy effort.

SECOND OPINION

MERV CROSS

Was a hard-tackling Rugby League forward for South Sydney, Eastern Suburbs and North Sydney in the early 1960s while he was studying medicine. Later he became a trail-blazing orthopaedic surgeon. Merv joined the board of the National Rugby League in 2000.

A ZANY GENIUS

I FIRST MET Brian during the 1960s when I was working out at City Tattersalls Club with the well-known trainer of sportsmen and women, George Daldry.

Back in those days all the football teams had an honorary doctor on their staff, but most had little knowledge of sports injuries. None were able to give any guidance on training methods, how stay fit and minimise injuries. It was all very unscientific. Most club doctors were GPs, in a bizarre twist, there were more than a few gynaecologists. Heaven forbid!

Someone told me about this bloke who was into sports medicine and I jumped at the chance to meet him. Our professional lives have been linked ever since. Brian can genuinely be described as the Father of Australia's Sports Medicine Physicians. He gave a real dignity to the profession.

In 1973 I accepted a fellowship in the United States to study how their surgeons treated sports injuries. Sitting on the sidelines at National Football League and college football matches opened my eyes. Back in Australia, I shared rooms in a surgery on Sydney's northern beaches with Brian and I decided to import Australia's first arthroscope (enabling a wide range of injuries to be treated in a non-invasive way through tiny incisions). At the time many of my fellow orthopaedic surgeons were against this new procedure, but Brian and his fellow rheumatologists gave me great support. They saw it as the way of the future. I'll never forget Brian's encouragement at that crucial time in my career. Today arthroscopy on sportsmen and women is common and the benefits are unquestioned.

While Brian Corrigan is well known for his efforts in sports medicine, he was also a superb rheumatologist who had a tremendous rapport with his patients. They swore by his treatment and stayed with him for life.

If I had to describe Brian in a few short words — zany, brilliant, a high achiever, but inclined to go off on tangents wherever his wonderful mind decides to take him.

A genius!

'Al Oerter slowly took off his neck brace and threw it to one side. The look on his face said it all, he was prepared to die, if that was needed, to win his gold medal.'

30. PROS AND CONS

THE WORD CON was originally American slang, short for confidence, referring to a confidence man, or con man for short, signifying conning, confidence trick or confidence trickster. People were conned into handing over their money or valuables, because the victims had unwisely placed their confidence in the person who was swindling them.

Australians have a reputation (surely unjustified) of being con men. The most famous case of an Australian con man was the fellow involved in the so-called Tichborne case. In 1854, the son of Lord Tichborne, heir to one of largest fortunes in England, went missing on a trip from South America to Australia. Many years later, a butcher from Wagga Wagga, Arthur Orton, claimed he was the missing son and returned with his wife to England to claim the inheritance. The elderly mother, Lady Henrietta, received him joyfully, but precious few others in the family did. Orton was arrested as an impostor and after a trial that lasted 120 days was sentenced to fourteen years in prison, still protesting his innocence. After his release in 1884, he admitted it had all been a con.

The ability to con received a big boost with the Internet and thousands of people received emails from Nigeria explaining how they could become incredibly rich without needing any great effort at all, just handing over the details of their bank accounts (including the PIN). The only people who became rich were the conmen in Nigeria.

The auctioning of sporting souvenirs over the Internet has also become so popular that people are now being conned into buying fake or unauthorised memorabilia. Johnny Raper would have had to have made a couple of hundred Test appearances if all the 'Raper' Test jumpers on offer were legitimate.

Over the past 40 years the meaning of the word has changed, so the more high-powered examples of conning are known by another American word, scam. These days, in Australia at least, conning does not have such an unkind or inconsiderate financial meaning. This applies especially on the sporting field. You commonly hear such statements as 'He is only conning himself', meaning someone is kidding themselves or 'He's trying to con you', meaning he is laying it on a bit thick. 'You're a con' is no worse an insult than the almost affectionate Australian exclamation 'You bastard'.

Conning in sport has been widespread for a long time, but it implies something different now. These days it is often regarded as being clever and much akin to gamesmanship. Sporting terminology now includes the expressions 'a psychological ploy' and 'mind games'.

Watch any football team, especially those from South America, try to con the referee into awarding them a penalty. The Brazilians in the 2002 World Cup, held 1–all by a determined Turkey, did exactly that. A theatrical dive in the penalty box conned referee Kim. The result, Brazil 2–1. A few minutes later, a Turkish player, Hakan Unsal, kicked the ball into the shin of Brazilian superstar Rivaldo, who fell hysterically clutching his face. Rivaldo should have been immediately sent off for over-acting, but Unsal was sent off instead. So bad was that decision that Rivaldo was fined after the game. He was unrepentant, claiming his con had been justified.

There are even instances of players trying to con their poor old doctor or coach into believing that an injury has recovered sufficiently for them to be able to return to the field. But we know better, don't we!

ONE OF THE first big sporting events I can remember as a child was the Davis Cup Challenge Round at Philadelphia in September 1939, played as German troops were marching into Poland. Harry Hopman was the Australian captain. His team was John Bromwich and Adrian Quist.

The Americans led two rubbers to nil after the first day. Australia then won the doubles rubber in a long, hard fought, five-set battle. On the

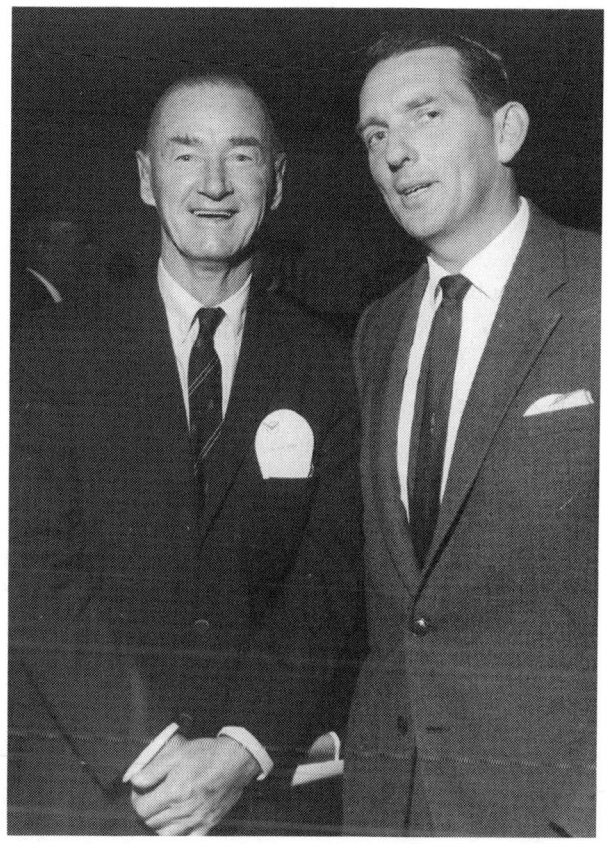

That old fox Harry Hopman knew just how to use reverse psychology to outwit his American opponents in the 1939 Davis Cup.
(BRIAN CORRIGAN'S COLLECTION)

third day, Quist, who currently holds the record for the most Davis Cup singles by any Australian, played the vital first game against Bobby Riggs. The match between the pair in the previous year's Challenge Round had ended with Riggs beating a tiring Quist. Hopman was determined there would not be a repeat performance. The score reached two sets to one, when normally the players would have a 10 minute rest. Hopman didn't want the break reasoning that if play stopped then Quist would become so stiff he would have great difficulty in starting again. In a stage whisper he let his American counterpart, Walter Pate, overhear a conversation suggesting how vital it was for Quist to have the rest period. Conned, Pate demanded that there be no break. Quist played on and won his rubber. Bromwich then won the fifth rubber easily and the Davis Cup was on its way to Australia. It was the first time any team had won after being down 2–0 on the first day.

No wonder Harry Hopman later became known as 'The Fox'.

OF ALL THE incidents I actually witnessed, two of my favourites involved Al Oerter and Shane Gould.

The American Alfred 'Al' Oerter is remembered for his remarkable feat of winning gold medals at four consecutive Olympics in the one event, the discus throw. Even more amazing, he did not hold the world record at the time of any of those four wins. He rarely held it. Thus at each of those Olympics he had to beat the current world record holder to win, and he also had to better his own Olympic record each time.

He was 20 years old when he first won, easily, at Melbourne in 1956. The following year he was involved in a near-fatal car crash, severely damaging some discs in his neck that never completely healed, leaving him permanently in a neck brace. Nevertheless, he competed in Rome in 1960 and won a gold medal by beating the then world record holder, fellow American Rink Babka, who ironically offered Oerter some advice during the competition that led to his record throw.

A week before the 1964 Tokyo Olympics, Oerter tore a lower rib cartilage. That doesn't sound much, but let me assure you it is an extremely

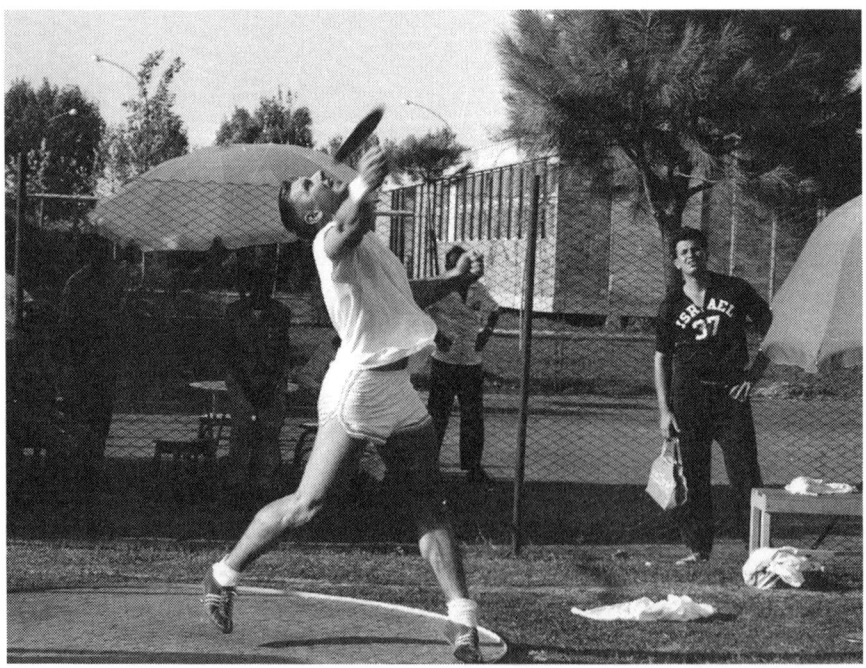

American discus thrower Al Oerter won four consecutive Olympic gold medals, from 1956 to 1968. He is shown here at the 1960 Rome Olympics. Oerter was the first to break the 200-foot (61-metre) barrier. (AAP IMAGE/SPORT THE LIBRARY/PRESSE SPORTS)

painful injury even in normal circumstances, let alone throwing a discus 60-odd metres in one massive burst. The American team doctors advised Oerter to forget about the competition, but he would have nothing of it. He threw 61 metres (just over 200 feet in the old measurements) to win gold.

To Mexico City in 1968. The world champion was Jay Silvester, who was expected to win easily. He qualified for the final with a massive throw, a new Olympic record and well past Oerter's best. The final was delayed an hour due to rain and this didn't help Silvester's nerves. Midway through the final, Oerter, who had been trying to throw while wearing his neck brace, was well behind. Then he stood up, turned to face Silvester and in a deliberate gesture, while still staring at him, Al Oerter slowly took off his neck brace and threw it to one side. The look on his face said it all, he was prepared to die, if that was needed, to win his gold medal with this next throw. He hurled the discus further than he had ever done before, once again in a new Olympic record of 64.78 metres. He shattered the morale of Silvester and the others. Well and truly conned, they fell apart, all finishing a long way behind. The runner-up was Lothar Milde with a throw 1.7 metres less than Oerter. Silvester could only manage fifth place.

SHANE GOULD WAS a truly great swimming champion and was the first woman to break Dawn Fraser's longstanding 100m freestyle world swimming record. Shane had set the new world's best in January 1972 at North Sydney pool. Her attempt at the record had attracted so much media hype that an estimated 2500 to 3000 fans were turned away after the 'house-full' signs had been raised.

Shane was a 15-year-old schoolgirl when she went to the 1972 Munich Olympics. A year before she had held the world record for every freestyle swimming event from 100 metres to 1500 metres. Her 1500 metres record of just over 17 minutes would have won a gold medal in the men's event in 1960 and 1964. There was huge psychological pressure, with the hopes of all Australians on her in Munich. She also carried a huge physical load having to swim fifteen times in eight days.

The mind games began as soon as she entered the swimming pool with the Americans wearing T-shirts that read, misquoting Shakespeare not once but twice: 'All that Glitters is not Gould'. Shane won her first race, the 200m individual medley, swum less than half an hour after her heat of the 100m freestyle. Gould's backstroke and breaststroke legs were average, but she did well in the butterfly leg and stormed home in the freestyle to take the gold in world record time from the 13-year-old East German, Kornelia Ender.

The following evening it was the 100-metres freestyle final. Gould was well behind at the turn, but despite another storming finish she could not overhaul Americans Sandra Nelson and Shirley Babaschoff. It was Shane's first loss in a freestyle event in two years. Next night came the 400-metres freestyle final. Gould gave no one a chance, beating Novella Calligaris of Italy by 3 seconds. Gould sliced 2.2 seconds off her own world record and 5.1 seconds off the Olympic best for a new mark of 4 minuntes 19.44 seconds.

Shane managed a day off before the race she had really set herself to win, the 200-metres freestyle. Lined up against her in the final were the current world record holder, Shirley Babashoff, and two other top Americans (as was allowed in those days). As Shane waited for the starter's pistol, the tension was unbearable. One American swimmer

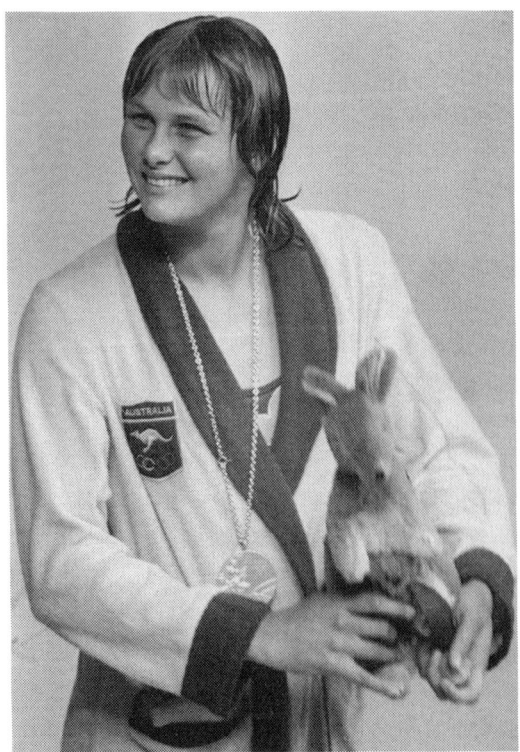

Even though she was only fifteen when she won her medal haul at the 1972 Munich Olympics, swimmer Shane Gould easily stood up to the pressure and mind games of her American medal rivals. (AAP IMAGE/SPORT THE LIBRARY/ PRESSE SPORTS)

deliberately broke to increase the pressure and make Shane wait a bit longer. As the American girl came out of the water, she had a surreptitious look around at Shane to see how greatly this had affected her. Shane, young as she was, had worked it all out and was sitting looking relaxed with knees crossed, attending to her fingernails. She then pretended to see someone she knew in the stand and gave a big wave. Shane had beaten the Americans at the conning game before she had even dived into the pool. She set up a huge lead in the first 100 metres. Babashoff cut it back a bit, but was well beaten at the finish as Shane carved almost a second and a half off the American's world record.

The next day Gould, feeling the effects of a chest infection (a cold is a medical emergency at the Olympics) and the strenuous program, finished second to American Keena Rothhammer in the 800-metres freestyle. Gould's final medal tally was three golds, one silver and one bronze. She was the only woman to have won three golds in individual events at an Olympics (each of them in world record time). She became the most successful Australian at any single Olympics, and that clever conning contributed.

SOMETIMES GAMESMANSHIP CAN all go horribly wrong. During the 1960s, the Manly Rugby League team was playing South Sydney one night when the young Manly second row, Billy Bradstreet, was suddenly propelled out of the scrum and was lying flat on his back, eyes shut. Bradstreet subsequently played one Test for Australia, but at that stage had not been in the first-grade team for very long. As I was attending to him I was swearing away out loud, asking why the referee didn't even award a penalty against South's John Sattler, one of the really hard men of League, and who was the obvious culprit.

Bill sat up, shook his head and told me he was all right. I went back to my seat, still grumbling about why the referee had done nothing. The next scrum that went down, Billy again came shooting out, blood streaming all over his face. He was carted off and I started to stitch up the big gash in his head, screaming even more about the refereeing.

'No, Doc,' mumbled Bill. 'Satts didn't hit me the first time. I was only conning the referee, trying to get Satts sent off. He sure got me the second time.'

Footballers certainly learn quick!

THEN THERE WAS this guy, no names no pack drill, who everybody regarded as a real pest. And with good reason because he was. He was always hanging around the Australian cricketers asking for any tales or secrets, which he swore he would never repeat. As soon as he found out some snippet of gossip he would quickly find someone, hopefully someone in the media, with whom he could share his newfound knowledge. He was doing that one night during a Test when the umpires were having dinner. They were not at all impressed with him, but told him one small fact on condition he never ever told anyone.

'You have my word of honour.'

Next day, one of the umpires raised his finger when the first wicket fell, and both umpires walked quickly towards each other and started warmly congratulating one another. Alan McGilvray, the cultured voice of ABC cricket, commented that this was a strange thing, something he had never seen before on a cricket field.

Our friend, who was in the ABC broadcasting box, piped up repeating what he'd been told the night before — 'That was the hundredth decision they have made together since they've been in Test Cricket.'

'Well, I didn't know that, what an interesting and unusual statistic,' said McGilvray and immediately broadcast this.

Of course, the umpires had made it all up and there was hell to pay when McGilvray found out he had been conned. That was definitely the last time the umpires were ever again bothered by the pest.

'Dame Margot told me that every morning when she woke up she would be in agony, but would force herself to perform at the barre every single day until her feet warmed up.'

31. DAME MARGOT AND SIR BOBBIE

FOR A WHILE I was the medical officer for the Australian Ballet, a job that I thoroughly enjoyed. One of the fascinating things was the incredibly hard work dancers would put in. Their degree of fitness was much greater than any football player I had ever known, and they would battle on through painful injuries, sometimes when I would have thought they would have been better off resting. I became firm friends with some of the dancers, like Dame Margot Fonteyn and Marilyn Jones.

Dame Margot was probably the greatest ballerina in history, the one against whom all others are measured. She was born in England in 1919, real name Peggy Hookham, and spent some of her childhood in China. When she was 14 she auditioned successfully for the Sadler's-Wells ballet, making her debut in 1934 as a snowflake in *The Nutcracker*. By the age of 26 she became prima ballerina with the Royal Ballet at Covent Garden. She established herself as an international star with a triumphant debut on the Royal Ballet's opening night in that city in 1949.

In 1956 she married Dr Roberto Arias, a Panamanian delegate to the UN. This led to some incredible incidents including one when she was arrested in Panama after her husband had been involved in an attempt to overthrow the government. He later became a quadriplegic after an assassination attempt in 1964.

Margot formed a wonderful dance partnership in 1962 with the younger Rudolph Nureyev, who had defected from the Soviet Union.

I first met her in about 1970 when she was performing in Sydney. We seemed to get on very well together. I sensed that everyone who met her asked the question: 'When are you going to retire?' After all she was a veteran in an industry that favoured young women. I studiously avoided any mention of retirement.

Her medical problem was with her feet. Dame Margot told me, and I most certainly believed her, that every morning when she woke up she would be in agony, but would still force herself to perform at the barre every single day until her feet warmed up. She had always refused any form of analgesics fearing they would slow her down. She was so beautiful and so delicate that I wondered how she kept going with such a cheerful disposition. She was a mighty determined lady.

Every night before going on the stage she would have to warm her feet up before her performance. She asked me to come and visit her in her dressing-room. Could I help with warming them up? Could I come to see her every night? I was amazed at how painful her feet were and wondered just how much damage she was doing to them by pushing herself so hard. I suggested we get an X-ray to assess the damage. She was completely opposed to this, saying she had never had her feet X-rayed because she was terrified at what sort of arthritis they would reveal. I thought it also might have been more of a superstition than anything else. Since I was getting on so well with her, I insisted and told her I couldn't treat her without an X-ray. I must admit I also had an ulterior motive for this, I was mighty curious to see just what state her feet were in. I got around it by saying we would get an X-ray, but I wouldn't show it to her or even discuss it with her. It was just to help my diagnosis. She agreed. The bony changes were even worse than I had anticipated, but, as promised, we never talked about the results.

She did talk about a lot of other things in her life. She told me her two great loves were dancing and her husband. She explained how seriously she took her marriage vows. This showed just what a great lady she was, because there were so many stories floating around about his repeated infidelity.

Dame Margot eventually told me how grateful she was that I never asked about a possible retirement. She did retire after that 1970 trip to Australia and went to live in seclusion in Panama with her husband. Before she left, she gave me an autographed photo of herself. With great modesty I can tell you that she wrote on it: 'Doctor Corrigan, you are the greatest!'

Dame Margot was one of the finest people I ever met.

THE LEGENDARY AUSTRALIAN ballet star Sir Robert Helpmann came to see me one day, resplendent in a pale blue velvet suit with a fur collar and an expensive dress shirt.

'Good afternoon, Sir Robert.'

'Oh, please, you *must* call me Bobbie,' he insisted.

'OK, Bobbie, call me Brian. What seems to be the problem?'

It appeared he had injured a lower rib cartilage.

'I'll show you,' he said, with a beaming smile. And with that he jumped to his feet, stripped naked, dropping all his finery onto the floor where he stood, and repeated, 'Watch. I'll show you!'

He then leaped across the room as graceful as a fawn. As he landed he grabbed his lower ribs, emitting a long drawn out and dramatic 'OOOH!!' Before I could say anything, he turned around and leaped once again into the air back to his original spot, with the same result. 'OOOH!!'

I was fascinated, to say the least, as both he and his appendage went flopping about from side to side in the breeze.

'Could you repeat that, if you do not mind, Bobbie?'

'Certainly, not a problem.' And off he went once more, cavorting across the room. Same result.

'Do you think you should see that one more time, Brian?' I can be a real bastard sometimes. The thought did cross my mind. I could have kept him repeating it for ages.

Instead I said: 'No thanks, Bobbie, I think I have seen more than enough. You might as well get dressed now'.

He picked all his beautiful clothes up from the floor and pranced out of the room.

STRIKE ME LUCKY!

Mo was one of the greatest names in Australian entertainment. An acclaimed comic, Mo was born Harry van der Sluys (sometimes written as the Anglicised Vander Sluice) in Adelaide in 1892. He wanted to be on the stage from his childhood days.

Harry took the stage name Roy Rene, from a vaudeville character he played and a French clown, while he was touring New Zealand in 1912 with a vaudeville troupe. Around this same time he added the stage makeup that was to become his trademark for the rest of his life — a white face mask with black beard. With this he became a caricature of a hooked-nose Jewish stereotype that these days would not be countenanced, too politically incorrect, even for Mo. The Mo part of his name came from possibly the most famous of all the characters he played in vaudeville, Mo McCackie, a clown. In 1914, he formed an incredibly successful partnership with fellow-comedian Nat Phillips. As *Stiffy and Mo* they entertained Australian audiences for the next 14 years, first with the Fuller Revue Company and then on the Tivoli circuit. The partnership continued until Phillips died in 1932.

After World War II, and before the arrival of television, Mo had a most successful radio show, *McCackie Mansions*. Many of his catchphrases — notably 'Strike me lucky' and 'Cop this young Harry' — became part of the Australian vernacular. His forte was innuendo and, after telling one of his suggestive stories, he would spit and splutter, 'Oh, you filthy beasts' to insult the audience who were laughing their heads off.

I first saw Roy Rene as a patient in 1954 after he suffered a series of heart attacks that left him somewhat incapacitated. He was still as funny then as he had been on the stage (his last stage show was *McCackie Mo-Ments* at Brisbane's Cremorne Theatre in 1949–50).

He had a garage crammed full with bottles of grog, mainly very expensive liqueurs as I recall. He knew he could never get through it all before he died, especially as he wasn't supposed to drink, so he would have many of his former theatre cronies around every Sunday morning to make some sort of dint in it. He would also invite me and I especially used to love listening to their stories, usually the bitchy ones about other actors.

One Sunday morning someone suggested that Evie Hayes was as good as Ethel Merman in *Call Me Madam*.

'Yeth, yeth, you're right,' said Mo, with his trademark lisp. 'One gets many thousands of dollars a week on the Broadway stage and the other a few hundred pounds a week on the Sydney stage. But yeth you must be right, she *is* better.'

I particularly loved the story of how Mo received a letter from the Governor. His Excellency had said something along the lines of 'your art is an important expression of the Australian ethos'.

'Gor blimey!' said Mo. 'I hope that ith a compliment.'

He had a severe attack one night and I was called to see him. He lay on the bed with his eyes closed, the room was in semi-darkness. His devoted wife Sadie Gale and their son and daughter were by his side. Soon after there was a knock on the door, his brother had arrived from Melbourne.

He clasped Mo's hand and whispered, 'Harry, can I get you anything?' Mo shook his head. Sadie was crying and it was all so dramatic I thought I would burst into tears, too.

'I've brought a bottle of champagne with me, maybe just a little sip?'

There was an almost imperceptible nod of the head. Then, as his brother was tiptoeing out of the room, Mo suddenly sat bolt upright in bed and called out to the departing figure, 'And none of that cheap pith. Make sure you've brought French Champagne.'

He died not long afterwards, on 22 November 1954, aged 63.

These days Roy Rene is remembered by the annual Mo Awards for excellence in the entertainment industry, but no performance could ever have compared with Mo's own that night.

'Their favourite tales were about some of their friends,
"brilliant journalists" who drank themselves to death,
one aged only 30.'

32. A MAD, MAD WORLD

IN MY TRAVELS over the years I have ended up in many unusual places and circumstances. A few of the incidents are worth sharing.

Pamplona, a small university town in Basque territory in a corner of northern Spain at the foot of the Pyrenees, is famous for its annual Running of the Bulls. After his visit there in 1924, Ernest Hemingway immortalised this celebrated event in his book *The Sun Also Rises*. It was one of his masterpieces — the story of expatriate American and British people from the lost generation after World War I, who partied their way from Paris to Pamplona, living their lives to excess.

The Running of the Bulls is (or it may be more accurate to say it was) a religious festival held for the past six centuries to celebrate the feast of San Fermin, the patron saint of winemakers, who was martyred in the town in the third century by being roped to a bull and dragged through the streets. The fiesta starts in the second week of July with a bullfight at the end of each afternoon. Then the party goes on for eight days, ending with the last bullfight on the Sunday night. The Basques, who seemed friendly, open, hard-drinking, tough people, belong to a club, or 'pena', symbolised by their traditional white uniform with red scarves knotted in front of the chest and thrown over one shoulder. One strange thing, for all the huge crowds and all the drinking, I never saw any fights or violence while I was there.

Bullfighting is certainly not everyone's cup of vino. Some are delighted, most are disgusted; some see it as an art, most see it as a barbarous exhibition; some say how incredibly brave, others say how unbelievably foolhardy. Only the Spanish and Portuguese now watch (and love) bullfighting, but there was a time when the fights were performed from the Mediterranean to the Far East.

This highly ritualised activity had its origins as a religious ceremony when, in ancient times, the bull was worshipped as being sacred, as a god. Its sacrifice and blood letting was considered part of the life/death/rebirth cycle described in Sir James Fraser's classic *The Golden Bough*. The blood symbolically fertilised the earth to allow the next harvest to grow.

It is virtually impossible to describe the scene at Pamplona. It is much worse than the Munich beer fest, for in the Bavarian capital usually people have a place to go to and sleep off their drinking excesses. In Pamplona, the tiny town is inundated with visitors, most of them have no place at all to sleep. They just fall down where they are or where they pass out, or they head to the local plaza or the park, nicknamed 'The Park Hotel'. Apart from the Basques, hordes of people from every country on the globe, drinking mainly cheap red wine from gourds, pack the narrow streets. At times, it can be virtually impossible to get through, the human traffic just does not move. Dancers dressed in bright colours surround the bands, whose musicians bang loudly and interminably on their drums, not caring about their own or anyone else's hangover or eardrums. The drinking is ferocious, it's the only time in my life I have been frightened of alcohol. And it goes on non-stop.

I travelled to Pamplona in 1981 with a friendly group of about 20 British journalists. It was an annual pilgrimage for them. Some of them had been going there for 20 years or more. They dropped their belongings in the small four-bedroom hotel they always rented, changed and did not return for about a week. Their favourite tales were about some of their friends, 'brilliant journalists' who drank themselves to death, one aged only 30.

One day, straight after the morning festivities, some of the group went to the Tres Reyes, the one upmarket hotel, for breakfast. A veteran member of the group ordered two ice buckets full of gin and tomato juice. He explained the tomato juice was because it was healthy. Just as the Spanish waiter was putting them on the table, he said, 'And another two, please.'

The waiter hesitated, staring in disbelief.

'That's the problem with the Spanish, they just don't understand serious drinking,' the journo explained.

I can't remember if we had our bacon and eggs or not, probably not.

One night, we were having dinner on a long trestle table in a restaurant, when a man and a woman who had recently met were overcome by lust and decided to do something about it there and then under the table. Nobody batted an eyelid. The pair emerged about 10 minutes later, with smiles on their faces, and rejoined the dinner party.

Every morning dead on (no pun intended) eight o'clock the mayor of the town would fire a rocket to start the day and seven or so bulls would come charging out of their corrals. Their ultimate destination was the stadium, the Plaza de Toros, approximately 2 kilometres away. They first had to race up a rather tricky steep hill. Then they would charge, hopefully in single file, through the narrow cobblestoned, often slippery streets, through the main drag, the narrow street called Estefeta, with balconies hanging above the turmoil (my favoured spot).

People pack the streets, the vast majority of them either trying to find a doorway or a niche in a wall in which to squeeze themselves, trying to dispossess any other onlooker already there, or standing pressed against the wall, stomach in and with both hands over their genitals. Or else close to the 6 foot wooden barricades, so they can rapidly jump over them.

The name 'running with the bulls' refers to the aim of running besides the bull, or more specifically 'on' the horn of the bull. It differs from 'running of the bulls' or corrida. The Corrida de Toros is the bullfight that takes place each afternoon in the bullring.

Some people start running as soon as they see the bulls approaching, but stay as close to the wall as they can manage. The brave, experienced participants run beside the bull, next to ('on') the horn, armed with a rolled-up piece of paper, and those that do this are suitably acknowledged. This is extraordinarily dangerous because the bull only has to toss its head a fraction to inflict horrible damage. It is not humanly possible for anyone to run as fast as a full-sized, cranky bull, travelling determinedly at approximately 50 kilometres per hour. It is only for a relatively short time, at best, that a runner can keep up. The greater danger lies in somebody slipping over on the wet streets. With people running everywhere as fast as they can and looking over their shoulders it is easy for several to fall right over the fellow who has slipped.

If the bulls keep running straight, playing follow-the-leader, as mostly happens, this is not such a huge problem. Should one or two become lost or separated from the herd, there is huge danger to anyone nearby, wherever they may be trying to hide, as the bull turns around blindly or tries to get back to where he has come from.

The next hazard comes at the entrance to the stadium where a bottleneck forms as the bulls and runners are herded into the stadium. When they all get in, the stadium is packed with cheering, drunken people in the stands, and hundreds of people, even more drunk than the spectators, running around at ground level trying to act like matadors. Madness! Finally, the bulls are steered into their corrals by professionals, ready for slaughtering at that night's bullfight.

Afterwards, everyone (Spaniards and tourists alike) retires to the main square, the Plaza de la Constitution, and proceeds to drink the cheap red wine until eight o'clock the next morning, when the cycle is repeated. The favourite drinking hole is the Café Iruna (Iruna is Basque for Pamplona), popularised by Papa Hemingway (a claim that could be made in most drinking holes across Europe, apparently). I soon found out that almost everyone boasted about how they had been running that morning, most of them right on the horns of the bull. And more seemed to have done it as the day wore on. Who could challenge the claims? After all, everybody else had his head down at the time.

Why would anyone do it? Indeed, why would anyone even want to do? Machismo (a peculiarly Spanish concept probably best translated as steroid madness) is the most likely explanation. After all, women are officially discouraged from running. There is no doubt there is a huge buzz in running it and the few who actually do run on the horn are extraordinarily brave people.

I could not run because I had torn my Achilles' tendon and could hardly walk, let alone run. Even without the injury, I never had any intention of running. But like every one else who says that, one becomes caught up with the mass hysteria and alcoholic haze, and ends up 'running', even if that means just getting on to the street as the bulls whiz past.

I'm mighty glad I experienced the Pamplona festivities, although I have never had the urge to do it again.

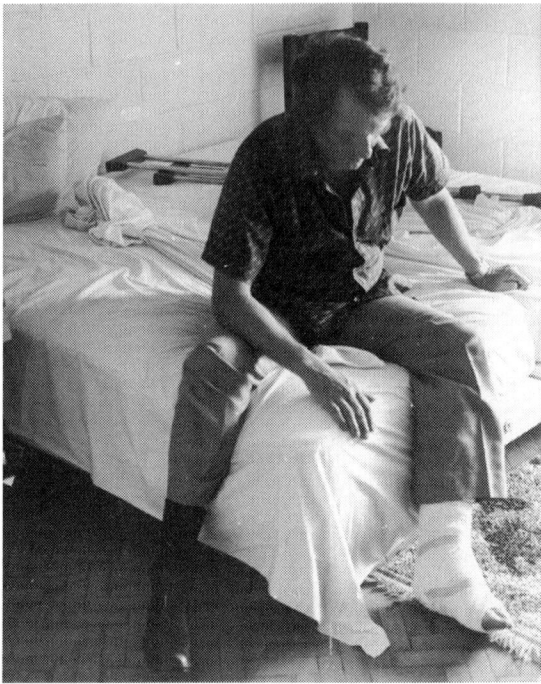

A torn Achilles tendon that shortly afterwards underwent surgery might have stopped me running with the bulls at Pamplona.
(BRIAN CORRIGAN'S COLLECTION)

IN 1973, CHINA was still a closed, isolated and mysterious country, although two years earlier the Communist authorities had instigated their new 'ping-pong diplomacy' in which they suddenly invited the US table tennis team to visit the country, the first Americans to be allowed in since 1949.

For a very long time I had wanted to go there, not least because I was interested to learn about acupuncture. Nothing was being taught about acupuncture in Western medicine and back then it was dismissed as a quack treatment. The other reason I wanted to go was to see how the so-called 'barefoot doctors' worked. There was a severe shortage of trained doctors away from the main city centres in China and Chairman Mao had village peasants trained to take a role in primary medical care.

At that time I had a real character as a patient. He was a South African named Sam Meyer, long since dead following a coronary occlusion. He gave me a present of some beautiful glasses and when I asked where they came from, he explained they were from China. The next question was inevitable. How did he get them out of there?

Sam told me a story that, at first, I had trouble believing. He said he was a South African spy who made regular visits into China under the cover of a salesman, selling things the Chinese needed. He didn't divulge what these products were and I felt it prudent not to ask. After a while, I did ask him how I could get into China, too. His reply was matter of fact. No problem at all. He wrote out a long, flowery letter, which I copied. It explained how China was one of the peace loving nations of the Pacific and how I would like to observe such things as their culture and learn about acupuncture. This letter was to be sent to an address in Beijing.

I really did not have too much faith in getting an answer. Sure enough, about two months later, a letter arrived. It requested I deposit $AUD60 into the Bank of China in Beijing. I immediately imagined lots of Chinese people running around with my cheque for $60 and no account to deposit it into. I sent it off anyway. It ended up being the total cost of my trip to China. Again to my surprise, I soon received a letter with instructions to board the train in Hong Kong for Canton (as it was then known) in about two months' time.

I booked a flight and arriving in Hong Kong, I was invited to stay with a wealthy American couple, Jim and Irene Latendresse, friends Monica and I had made when Jim was working in Sydney. They lived in Hong Kong, very close to the Peak, in splendid isolation from the crowds below. They were absolutely horrified that I was going to China at all. There was even more consternation when they had been told that the Chinese people did not have anything to eat, so I could starve to death on my four-day trip. When they realised I was determined to go, Irene told her amah to make me a large packet of sandwiches to take with me.

I arrived at the station in Hong Kong with no ticket and no specific identification except for the letter and the sandwiches. A man came up and showed me to a seat. I was easily identified as I was the only Westerner on the train. When I arrived at the border I got off the train and crossed a bridge on foot into China. I was feeling quite isolated, apprehensive and hungry. I began to wonder if I should start on my pile of sandwiches. I was met on the other side of the bridge, taken to a nearby building and led into a room where there was a table laden with a huge Chinese meal, more than I could ever hope to eat. I realised I was not going to starve in China. I was then taken to a train and put in a whole carriage all to myself.

As the train approached Canton, I started to feel a little anxious about what was to happen. Sure enough, just as the train was pulling in, a

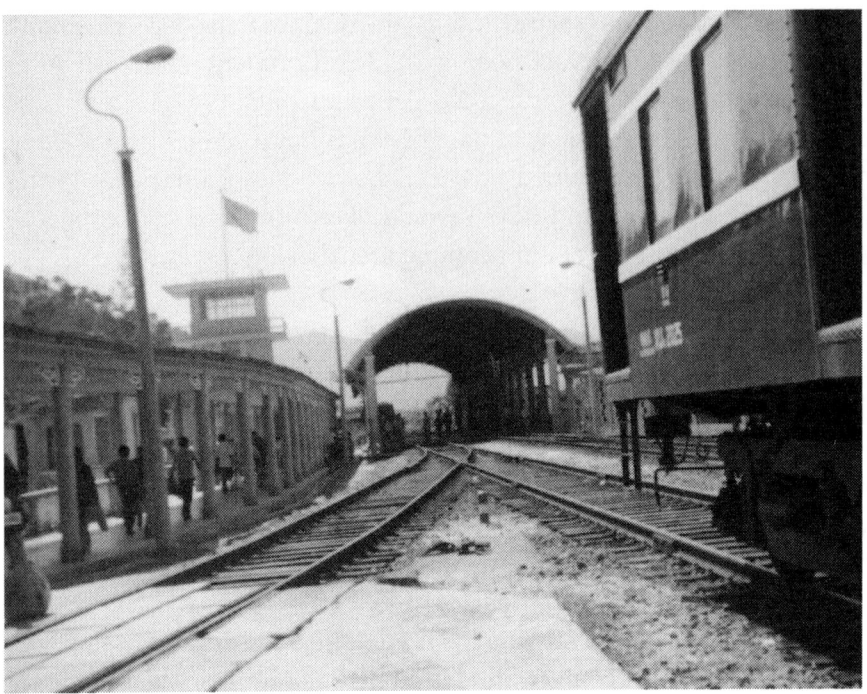

China really was a new frontier when I managed to visit that isolated and mysterious country in 1973 to study acupuncture. The train pulling into Canton.
(BRIAN CORRIGAN'S COLLECTION)

Chinese man appeared and asked a question that would be repeated many times over before I left, 'Where is your delegation?' He was more than reluctant to believe there was no delegation, only myself, and I was later to learn it had been expected that the first visitors would be in groups and delegations. He finally took me to the incredibly ugly, Russian-built Friendship Hotel, where another large meal was laid out.

The following day I was taken to see an operation performed under acupuncture. The surgeon had trained for many years in America and spoke excellent English. The long operation to remove a kidney stone was most impressive as the patient remained conscious the whole time. When the surgeon removed the stone, he held it up triumphantly to show the patient. He then held the stone against the X-ray to show him where it had been. What an excellent psychological ploy! His patient then got off the table and jumped up onto a trolley to be wheeled to the recovery ward.

After the operation, I was taken to a room with the surgeon and his assistants, including an interpreter, lined up on one side of a table, while

I lined up on my own on the other side. I realised I was expected to give a speech and ask questions through the interpreter. The surgeon suddenly could not speak English, only Chinese. I was most sincere in telling them that I was very impressed with everything, that the patient did not seemed to have any pain at all during the long operation, but did he feel pain afterwards?

'Of course he does,' said the surgeon via the interpreter.

'What do you do about it, then?'

'They give him an injection of pethidine, of course,' the interpreter told me. I didn't expect that. They explained how it was much cheaper to give an injection than use the manpower and time involved in administering more acupuncture.

THE NEXT DAY, I was taken to a village to meet the local 'barefoot doctor'. It was difficult to communicate, even though I did have an interpreter with me. The doctor had a very full waiting room and was administering acupuncture to the lower leg of his first patient. After the treatment that patient, who seemed pleased with the result, bowed to the practitioner and left.

The interpreter asked me whether I had any questions.

'Yes, may I have a go at the acupuncture with the next patient?'

The acupuncturist made signs to signify that it was impossible. I wasn't qualified.

'Fair enough,' I thought.

However, the doctor signalled he would be most pleased to demonstrate on me if I had any medical problems.

I couldn't think of any. It didn't matter, he would demonstrate acupuncture on my leg. Roll up your trousers!

He pulled down a rusty old tin holding even older and rustier needles, took one out and wiped it on a rag as a sop to sterilisation. It was too late to back out now. I was worried enough about the sterility of the needle, but even more conscious of the large nerve in my leg he seemed to be aiming for. He stuck the needle in the muscle of my lower leg, away from the nerve, and started twirling it for quite some time.

The interpreter explained, 'You will feel your leg go numb in a short time and it will be difficult to walk.'

'Nonsense', I thought to myself. After all, I knew he was nowhere near the nerve. With that, my leg started to go numb and when I tried to stand up, my lower leg felt weak and I had to drag my foot. The interpreter thought it was immensely funny watching me trying to walk, but said it would wear off in a few hours.

I spent some hours there and what impressed me most was that the doctor spent a long time checking the patient's pulse, all the time talking and having great rapport with each patient.

When I got back to the hotel, there on the bed, was the unopened bag of sandwiches from Hong Kong, which I had thrown in the bin that morning. As I was going to a huge farewell banquet that night, I threw them away again.

Next morning, the interpreter and I arrived at the train station. As the train started to pull out, a man from the hotel arrived, and ran along the platform shouting, and handed me a parcel — the bag of sandwiches. I eventually returned the unopened bag of stale sandwiches to Irene. She explained how she and Jim had been convinced they would never see me again. To celebrate my return they offered to take me out that night for a Chinese meal. I explained diplomatically that while I really loved Chinese food, could I possibly have a steak?

IN 1970, MY colleague Dr Dave Codey and I were invited to go on a lecture tour around New Zealand. Our last point of call was the university town of Dunedin. We arrived a bit early for our last lecture, so we decided to go and have a beer. I have to tell you that Dave was a fairly solidly built ex-Rugby Union representative player who liked a beer or five. The pub we found was rather seedy-looking, but handy. When we walked in, we were immediately greeted by a deathly silence and glares from the 10 or so customers seated around the wall. It was an eerie feeling.

Well, so what, we were going to be out of there shortly, we thought, and went up to the bar to order our beer. Before we had been served, the largest and toughest-looking man the group, obviously the leader, came up, stood in front of us and said in a menacing tone, 'You are DS'.

We had no idea what he was talking about and tried to explain that to him. We obviously weren't getting through because he repeated the same comment, 'You are DS'.

'Look, we truly do not understand what that means. We are Australians,' (strange, but that did not seem to cut much ice with him or any of the group). 'And …' I didn't finish the sentence as he cut in belligerently, 'We do not believe you.' With that his assembled mates made acquiescing sorts of noises, although still no one else had spoken.

It really was looking nasty, especially when someone closed the hotel doors. With that our man pulled out a pair of dice and said, 'We will ask the dice.' And he rolled them out on the bar.

He immediately relaxed and broke into something I thought could have even been a smile. He explained that the dice believed us. Now everything was all right. The menace went out of the room. He said the beer was on him and the hotel doors were re-opened. We could explain to everyone's satisfaction who we were and why we were there.

It turned out that the man who had confronted us was a 'dice man'. He explained how he lived his whole life by what the roll of the dice told him to do. We found that to be unbelievable, until Luke Rhinehart's entertaining book *The Dice Man* came out a short time later. Apparently there was an outbreak of people who followed the instructions of the dice implicitly, even if, as with the hero in the book, their life was ruined.

Everything was now going well, even though our newfound friend had the disturbing habit of rolling the dice every time there was any sort of decision to be made.

'What was DS?' we could now ask.

'Drug Squad,' came the reply.

'What would have happened to us if the dice hadn't believed us? Would your mates have killed us?'

Silly question, he seemed to be thinking, but he answered, 'Oh no, they would not have killed you. But they would have nearly killed you.' Very comforting!

The dice man and his mates insisted that we were not to buy any beer, that they would do all the shouting (I'm not too sure if the dice had decided that or not). He told us, quite frankly, he was a drug dealer. One reason he hated the Drug Squad so much was they would come and confiscate his drugs and then re-cycle them out into the street. It was all very fascinating stuff and they kept buying us beers.

Eventually, and most reluctantly, we had to leave. By now we were late for our lectures … and not in the best of shape.

We never went back to that bar. The dice told us not to!

I WAS ONCE at a sports medicine meeting in New York, after which Monica and I were to fly to San Francisco where I was due to attend a rheumatology conference. We planned to get together with Ian Chappell and his wife, Kay, who were on a Qantas promotional tour. We were also to meet our daughter, Carolyn, who had just finished her nursing training and was flying in from Sydney. We arranged to all meet up at our hotel and then go to dinner on the Friday night.

The first hint of trouble came on the Friday when Monica and I arrived at the Sir Francis Drake Hotel. There was a most officious man behind the reception desk. This was, I must say, most unusual for an American hotel, where the staff normally fall over themselves to ensure guests enjoy their stay. This bloke reckoned we had no booking, despite us showing him documentation that confirmed we had booked ahead. Finally after much arguing and with great reluctance he agreed to give us a room.

The Chappells had said they would ring us at our hotel, as they had not been too sure where they would be staying, but there were no phone call from them.

Then came the real disaster — there was no sign of Carolyn arriving. As time ticked away, her two increasingly anxious parents contacted the airport. The plane from Sydney had definitely arrived several hours ago. We checked with Sydney. She had definitely left on that plane. We checked again with the lobby. No, no one with that name had booked in. We rang a Qantas pilot, Les Symons, who was a close friend. He checked with the purser on Carloyn's flight. The purser remembered her being on the plane and, in fact, had noticed that she was sitting next to a very strange-looking character. At this news Monica and I became even more concerned.

We decided we should contact the police, who arrived reasonably promptly. One was a big blond man, the other a small brunette woman both carrying all sorts of weapons. He seemed a very nice fellow, but she didn't say much as he dominated the conversation.

'Would you happen to have a Scotch?' was his first question. We gave him our bottle of duty free, which the two of them proceeded to work their way to the bottom of it.

Next question. 'I suppose you've checked all the hospitals and the morgue?'

No, we hadn't thought of that.

'I'll do it for you,' he offered. He made a call, explaining: 'We are looking for a young, white, Caucasian woman, missing, presumed (pronounced pre-zoomed) dead. Yes, I'll hang on.' The bottle was rapidly emptying.

Presumed dead? Oh, no! You can't possibly be serious. We both felt the life draining away. After a time, it turned out that Carolyn had not been admitted to any of these places.

'Look, that's all we can do,' he told us. 'You will have to contact the airport police, they will have jurisdiction in this case. You need the Sheriff of San Mateo. Except you won't be able to find him now, it's too late. He starts work at the airport at six o'clock in the morning.'

They finished the last of the Scotch and left. It was very late, but we could not sleep at all. All through that long night, we could hear sounds of police and ambulance sirens, each one like a knife plunging into our body.

Next morning, I caught a taxi to the airport and right on six o'clock was outside the office of the Sheriff of San Mateo. He said, not unkindly, 'Look, I get hundreds of these cases, and they always turn up OK. Don't worry, she's away some place screwing.'

'She may be away screwing,' I said, impugning my daughter's honour, but didn't have the time to argue that point. 'But I know she would have told us that's where she was.'

He shrugged his shoulders, 'Look, there is nothing I can do or tell you. You'll just have to wait.'

Crestfallen, I returned to the hotel. I thought I would contact the Australian Consul and see if he could help, but only received a recorded message informing me the Consulate was shut on a Saturday.

I went to the reception desk again wondering if they could help me find an emergency number for the Consul, but the same officious check-in man was on duty.

'Go around the back and check with the telephone operator,' he snarled. 'See if she can help?' So I went into the little office behind the desk, just in time to hear the operator say, 'Yes, Corrigan, connecting you now.' The room number she mentioned was not the one in which we were staying.

How could she put someone through to Corrigan when neither of us was in that room? I asked her if could I be connected to the room in question. And Carolyn answered. Unbelievable relief!

It transpired that we did have the correct booking in the first place, but our overbearing man at reception put us into another room. When Carolyn arrived, a different man on the desk put her into our original room which had been booked all the time. She was jet-lagged, didn't worry about us not being there, and thought we must be coming in later, so she went to sleep. Chappelli had rung us on the Friday night, but was told we hadn't booked in. He said he would ring again the next morning, and it was his conversation with the telephonist that I overheard.

There was a very tearful but most relieved meeting between the three Corrigans. Thanks to that awful man on the desk there had been all that angst for nothing.

'Every time the waves hit me I would go under, get a gutful of sea water, and surface just in time for the next big wave to smack me down again ... I was drowning!'

33. THE CRUEL SEA

MOST DROWNINGS IN Australia involve children aged one to four, usually at home, while swimming in pools or playing in bathtubs. This is despite safety precautions and rules in place to try to prevent this.

The number of adult drownings on this continent is also a concern. In 2002, there were 60 adult deaths by drowning, although according to the Australian Bureau of Statistics, the long-term trend in accidental drowning declined from 2 per cent of accidental deaths to less than 1 per cent now. This may have a lot to do with the wonderful job our volunteer lifesavers do.

Male deaths predominate by a margin of at least two to one with the most common age being 15 to 35, while most drownings take place in December and January when there are a quarter of all deaths, and the least number in May. Deaths in home pools and bathtubs are also becoming less common. There is a long list of causes of drowning, including falls into the water, surfboard riding and spear-fishing.

The one that always amazes me, and you'd think it was eminently avoidable, is being swept off the rocks while fishing, especially in big seas. In another older-age group, deaths occur while boating and it is most likely that alcohol plays a role.

Australians are now more or less growing up with a greater knowledge of the hazards of the water, but foreign tourists who do not understand the surf can be more of a problem, as they often do not recognise their limitations in the water. On a Sydney beach, two Japanese women tourists nearly drowned about 10 metres from the shore. One was knocked over by a wave, but couldn't swim and panicked. She also knocked over her friend who had gone to help her. She, too, panicked, struggled and the pair was lucky to be rescued.

There are also problems with diving into the water. I remember taking a German friend for a car trip to the country. It was a very hot day and we decided to strip off for a swim in a pleasant creek. I looked around expecting to see him wading in. To my horror, he dived in headfirst. If he had struck his head in the shallow water or one of the rocks he would be left a paraplegic for life.

Some years ago, we went on a January holiday weekend to Laurieton, a small, agreeable seaside village on the north coast of New South Wales. One afternoon, I had played cricket with my then 14-year old son, Dominic, and we decided to go for a long run along the beach. It was getting fairly late by the time we'd finished, and feeling fairly hot, we decided to go for a swim. This was a very poor decision for several reasons. In the first place, the beach was deserted and there were no lifeguards. We should have heeded the warning sounded when the Prime Minister, Harold Holt, drowned on a deserted Victorian beach in 1967, but the waves did look particularly inviting, and we were not thinking of any possible trouble.

At the time there was a long sandbank. We swam out to where the waves were breaking and were enjoying a pretty good surf for a while, with no problems. I came in on one wave but as I was wading out again, I could feel the sand shift and disappear from under my feet. I swam out to where Dominic was, conscious that we were in a rip. I told him not to talk, just to swim back to shore as fast as he could. I must have sounded convincing, because, for the first time in his life, he didn't argue, and headed off immediately. I stayed in the water to make sure he was all right.

A big wave came along and I thought I would try to ride it back. As I started to swim strongly for it — wham — I tore a tendon in my right shoulder. The pain was intense and I had to tread water as I couldn't use my arm at all for a few minutes. There was by now no sandbank at all and the rip was getting stronger. I should have gone with the rip, but I thought I could still get back, except that I could no longer swim strongly enough with my shoulder.

All of a sudden I was in very deep water. The waves, getting bigger and rougher all the time, were breaking over and engulfing me and every time they hit me I would go under, get a gutful of sea water and surface just in time for the next big wave to smack me down again. It was all happening so quickly; I couldn't see the shore, only the huge waves and the sky. I was getting weaker and suddenly realised that it would not take much for me to be unable to come up at all.

I was drowning!

At times like this your whole life is supposed to flash before your eyes. That did not happen, although two thoughts did. It was my birthday and I did think how stupid, nobody should drown on their birthday. The other was the relief I felt believing that Dommie had made it to the shore, although that turned out to be a mistake.

I seriously thought that it was the end. I'm gone. I knew I couldn't come up again after the next wave and waited for its arrival. Like a manna from heaven, a young fellow on a surfboard appeared beside me, and gestured for me to hang on to the board.

Dominic had also got into difficulty, and the young surfer, walking home along the beach carrying his board, had seen him. He went out to rescue him and was taking him back to the beach.

Dominic told him, 'My father is missing out there somewhere.'

'No way, no one else could be out there,' the surfer replied. But Dominic pleaded with him to return to have a look, and somehow he managed to find me.

The drama was not finished. The surfer fell off his board. I was left holding the board with one good arm and was not able to do much to help him get back on the board. He managed to grab the other side of it. I told him that if we both hung on to it, we would eventually get washed back to shore. Which we did.

Eventually, I lay exhausted on the sand and vomited up half the Pacific Ocean. I had narrowly missed out on becoming another statistic.

Lucky!

'The surgeon came in and said ... "You have a cerebral tumour. You've got about three months to live. You might as well have it operated on".'

34. A BRAIN TUMOUR

IN 1986, AGED 57, I developed a brain tumour, which on a malignancy scale of one to four, rated three. Up until that time, I had been feeling particularly well, particularly fit, was working hard and doubtless had delusions of being indestructible.

The first symptom was that I felt terrible when I woke up each morning. It's hard to explain what that means, but I didn't have any energy so that it was a struggle to get up and go to work. Some mornings I didn't want to get out of bed at all, although that invoked no sympathy in our household. In fact, I thought maybe I was imagining it or only being lazy, even though I still did have a feeling that something dreadful was happening to me. Once, I had to give an early morning lecture, but felt as though I hadn't slept for a fortnight. I received no sympathy for that either and it was a bit frustrating trying to explain it. The lousy feeling tended to wear off a bit during the morning and I might not have any great trouble for the rest of the day. I thought I couldn't go to a doctor and say 'I didn't feel well' with nothing else wrong with me.

After a short while I developed a funny feeling, like an absence or vagueness. In the middle of a sentence I would suddenly lose track of the word or thought I was having, only for a short time, then I would resume normally. I mentioned this to a few medical colleagues, but did not get too far with them either.

'What are you talking about, you've always been that vague, you've developed it into an art form,' was the usual reply.

Or they'd ask, 'Do you get these when you're busy?'

'Busy, I'm always bloody busy.'

'Oh well, that explains it. You put too much stress on yourself.'

I tried to ignore or cover up the symptoms. I still felt sure there was more to it than that, but there were no other symptoms, never any severe headaches, and when I did get headaches they did not seem to be increasingly more common, so what else could I do? The absences of the mind started getting more frequent, and working was starting to become a problem. I decided I definitely needed to have some investigations done and made an appointment to see a neurologist.

The same day I made the decision to seek help, I was taking a group of students on ward rounds when I became ill, sicker than I had ever felt. I asked my registrar, Michael Prowse, if he could take over, as I thought I should go home to bed. He took one look at me, said, 'There's no way you're going home', and he arranged a bed in the hospital immediately.

It was just as well, for he saved my life!

I can remember climbing into bed and thinking how white and cool the sheets were and how pleased I was to be there, because there was no way I could have driven my car home. I had a massive convulsion and lost consciousness. At least I did not know anything about the convulsion. It was later discovered that I had fractured 12 vertebrae and one tooth.

I came to early next morning in Intensive Care, panic-stricken, for I had a tube down my throat to assist my breathing after the heavy medication to stop the convulsions. I was half-conscious, but felt sure I was going to choke and couldn't communicate with anyone to tell them what was happening. It was a terrifying experience, and to this day, I can still feel the terror. I started roaring so loudly, still half-unconscious, that I woke Monica, who was sleeping outside.

An MRI investigation showed a tumour the size of an orange on the left side of my brain and I was admitted for immediate surgery. I felt pleased when I found that a friend, who had been in the same year with me at Sydney University and with whom I had worked at the same hospital, was to perform it. The surgeon came in and said three sentences in total: 'You have a cerebral tumour. You've got about three months to live. You might as well have it operated on.' And he walked away.

'Thanks a lot, mate.'

Now, strangely, I did not feel especially anxious or fearful about this. I am not too sure why, for worry and fear are, after all, natural reactions and I was never trying to act tough or disregard it. Maybe it was because there was no great degree of pain. Or maybe I relaxed because the diagnosis was no longer uncertain and at least something positive was being done. Most certainly, no one would ever want anything like this to happen, and I really am not stupid, but it was easy to deal with because there was no agonising decision to be made. There was only one answer: 'Yes, and how soon can the operation be done? Just do it.'

The surgeon did tell Monica and the children that if he could remove it all, I might be all right, although when they told me that I was not really comforted by the word 'if'. He also told them a few other things they didn't get around to telling me at that time. He warned them the tumour was located in a difficult area, very close to the pathway for my eye, and I was very likely to lose the sight in that eye. There was also a very good chance he would not be able to remove it completely. If so he would just sew me up again.

There were still a few more tests to be arranged, then on to the big day, although I don't remember much about it at all. I do remember coming out of the anaesthetic that night after the seven-hour operation and although still half-asleep, I realised that I could think. It was the most unbelievably comforting sensation, knowing I could think, even though I still could not talk or see. I lapsed back into sleep. As I became fully conscious, I recognised my family all sitting around the bed looking anxious, and was told that the news from the operation was very encouraging because the surgeon had removed the entire tumour. Great! I was given a sleeping tablet and awoke next morning in Intensive Care, feeling surprisingly well, with only a slight headache, and was told I was so well I could go back to the ward. I was out of hospital in a week and ready to go back to work in a month.

There was to be one complication; because of swelling in the brain, I had to take high dosage cortisone tablets to reduce it. Whenever I gave them to patients in a dose of, say, one to four tablets in a day, they would invariably look at me askance, and say, 'Are you trying to kill me?' I was on 24 tablets four times a day. That's right, 96 tablets a day. I felt like I was being poisoned and sure the doctors were trying to kill me. There was no arguing; there was so much swelling around the brain that I was in trouble. The tablets completely blew my mind; I felt extremely uptight and weepy and couldn't sleep. The only good thing was the realisation that these symptoms were due to the tablets and would ultimately disappear. Luckily, I responded quickly to them and the swelling was diminished. So I came off the high dose fairly rapidly, and started to feel all right again.

The nursing staff was fantastic. They could not have been bettered. How could anyone ever forget their dedication and care? Nurses are so criminally underpaid, the work they do is priceless.

WHAT THEN OF the future? If I only had a few months to live, there was not much point planning an extensive cruise to some exotic place or some similar experience. I would be far better off spending time with my wife, children and grandchildren.

I still had to undergo a lengthy and exhausting course of radiation therapy. That turned out to be worse than anything that had befallen me before. It was not that the staff members were not caring and helpful, because they most definitely were. A deep X-ray department is no place to sit on a cold winter morning among so many desperately ill patients, most with the look of certain death in their eyes. Nor did it help to have to climb up onto a hard table every morning and lie completely still with a broken back. I lost all my hair and wore a cap for some months. The loss of hair was no real concern to me, but I could see it might be a blow for a woman to lose hers.

The first few days back home, I felt so unbelievably sick and weak, I could hardly walk. I had made up my mind that on that first day home, I was going for a walk. I could hardly make one block and needed help from one of the kids. Next day, two blocks with one of them. Third day we tried a small hill and went all right, so after that I could go out on my own.

A well-meaning doctor friend turned up. He said he was worried about my attitude. How the hell did he know what my attitude was when I had not seen him in months? I told him thank you, but not to worry. I tell this story for a reason. A great help in the recovery process is the presence of well-wishers and friends, but they can also present a problem. They often tell patients about various treatments (often conflicting treatments) and offer advice (usually useless advice) they have heard or read or know about that cures cancer. The end result? The poor patient is left more confused than ever about what to do or think.

I have always been conscious of the fact that the mind is very powerful in the recovery process — a positive attitude is always essential and I was determined to work towards this, as a negative attitude would be a disaster. What do those words mean? Are they just a lot of words, a vague feeling that has different meanings to different people? How do you achieve a positive attitude? Does a positive attitude just mean a lack of a negative attitude? There is no single correct way to develop a positive attitude; it is a process, an inner belief that recovery is not only possible, but is going to happen. You must decide you want to get well, act as if you are going to get better, and have a plan for the future. You change the things you can change and don't become stressed about things you can't. This includes the cancer; get on with treatment and your life. Never be afraid of expressing your emotions. Cancer need not be a death sentence.

I also realised that it must be a great deal easier to feel positive if the problem is correctly diagnosed early than it would be for an advanced case. A positive attitude comes easier when a treatment plan is presented, or you are successfully operated on, rather than if lots of tests are required and the diagnosis still remains doubtful. Is there any evidence that a positive attitude does have any benefit, besides being just a nice gut feeling? Psychologists I ask can't give me a satisfactory answer to this or if there is any scientific evidence that it really works. To my mind the single most important factor, by a long way, in developing a positive attitude is the love and support you receive from your spouse and your family.

So what do you do? Do you take lots of vitamins? I felt sure multi-vitamins or supplements are grossly over-hyped, irrelevant if you are still eating a normal diet. Is meditation of any value, and how many people practise it properly? Could it really have any impact or long-lasting effect on immunological or hormonal systems? Who knows the answers?

Lots of people said I was brave. Was I brave? I honestly don't think so. It was just the hand I had been dealt and so that was the hand I had to play. I was very determined to get back to exercising and back to work as fast as I could, and I did. Although I was a bit wobbly, I was back at work in one month.

Recently, it has been recognised just how common depression can be in cancer patients. It plays a significant role in at least 25 per cent of cases, and can be treated successfully. Patients with depression and anxiety feel there is a real stigma attached to being depressed. They feel embarrassed, ashamed, and cannot or do not want to recognise it, discuss it, see a psychiatrist or psychologist. Other reactions such as guilt, grief, sadness, anger and blame are beyond discussion here. The answer is to be sure you see some health professional as early as possible and, most importantly, eschew the myriad of quack cures and the false hopes that are sold to the unwary. I was lucky enough not to have this problem, which can be a scourge of so many.

I never asked, 'Why me?' Some people tell me I got better because it was God's will. I can never understand that, since if that were the case, it surely would have been a great deal easier for Him and everyone else involved just to have not let it happen in the first place. If He is to get the credit for curing someone, surely He has to take the blame for causing it, and I don't think that gets us too far down the track.

The psychological and emotional response to a life-threatening illness, whatever it may be, has always been of great interest to me to see how people react and how this varies so much. Probably there are as many reactions as there are people.

One patient, a family friend of many years, used to drive me to distraction, not a nice thing to say, but true nevertheless. He would come to see me with a variety of illnesses, often minor, and would spend an hour or more asking what it was, how long before he would get better, what complications could there be and so on. All very reasonable questions, but he would ask them over and over, and then ring me the following day to ask me again. He came to see me one day looking dreadfully ill. It didn't take too long to determine he had cancer in his liver and needed to be admitted to hospital. I thought, how am I ever going to explain all this to him and how will he react? He never asked a question, never said a word. He died in hospital, painfully. I saw him almost every day, but he never once asked his wife or me what the diagnosis was or what was to happen to him.

Another patient had a widespread and very painful cancer. He was a Scot and said he would like to go to Scotland to see his relatives before he died. I thought he had little chance of getting there and back, especially with the problem of trying to control his pain. He was determined. On his return home, he told me he had no pain at all while he was in Scotland. His pain returned just after his plane landed at Mascot Airport and he died about one week later.

I had to have a brain scan every year, and did so diligently for 10 years. About that time, I felt a sudden severe pain in my head, which over the next couple of days became worse. This is it, I thought, my old enemy has returned. Then I remembered getting out of my car earlier, I suddenly twisted my neck, rather violently. The brain scan was once again normal and after physiotherapy fixed my neck and head pain, I decided I was cured of my tumour and needed no more scans.

Fingers crossed!

SECOND OPINION

SUE CORRIGAN

Is the daughter of Brian and a senior feature writer with the *Mail on Sunday* newspaper in London.

ROLL OVER BEETHOVEN

WE FIVE CORRIGAN kids are all very proud of Dad's career and his many achievements.

It's our mother Monica, though, who made much of this possible, I know Dad would be the first to acknowledge her. He's always relied very heavily on her support, organisational skills and hard work, keeping things running smoothly at home while he studied and worked and travelled. Dad was often absent when we were growing up, but Mum was always there, holding everything together for him, and for us.

Throughout my teens, we seemed to be constantly at Sydney Airport, farewelling Dad and various national sporting teams, or welcoming them all back again. It seems as though we drove up and down that old road through the suburb of Mascot, past all the rancid-smelling factories, a thousand times. Yet it left me with an abiding love of airports, the smell of aircraft fuel and departure boards with their exotic lists of cities all over the world just waiting to be explored.

In the days when Dad started travelling with sporting teams in the mid-1960s people just didn't jump on and off planes like they do today. International travel was still incredibly glamorous, and his comings and goings gave me a certain cachet with my school friends, who were always amazed how often he was out of the country. I got a big laugh in the speech I gave at my wedding reception when I thanked Dad for passing up the opportunity to attend the world mud wrestling championships in Zagreb to be with us. I bet some people there were not entirely sure whether I was joking or not.

Dad's passion for travel, sport and any sort of adventure reflects his passion for life in general. His enthusiasm for the things he loves is intense: classical music, words, books, ideas, cricket, medicine, exercise and the *Sydney Morning Herald*'s cryptic crosswords. There is also Dee Why beach and the view of the ocean from the house where he and Mum have lived since 1957. Sydney and Australia are also high on the list.

He's always been and still is, in a funny sort of way, young. He's remarkably non-judgmental and open to new ideas and experiences. In his late 60s, he took passionately to computers, even though he had a terrible struggle getting on top of the technology. I vividly remember in the early 1960s that he just loved the Beatles, which was not the sort of thing most parents of that era would admit to. He loved their music and even took us to the old Sydney Stadium for one of their concerts in, I think, 1964, when I would have been around 11. I was pretty impressed at the time by his modernity.

Dad and Mum gave great parties and always had tons of good friends. Dad loved dancing and Frank Sinatra. Most of all, though, he's always loved classical music, Beethoven in particular. He often took me to orchestral performances and was always explaining the various instruments. For several years, he drove us to our secondary school, which was some distance from home, and he'd always insist on us listening to classical music as we sat in the traffic jams. It was very annoying at the time, but I appreciate it now.

Dad also introduced me to politics and gave me a strong sense of social justice. He used to be a committed Labor Party supporter, in the days when political allegiances more acutely reflected people's sense of their class position, and everybody else we knew voted Liberal. I remember being taken to a polling station when I was very young (in my pyjamas) and asking him which party he was voting for. When he said the Labor Party, I asked him why. He said, 'Because they try to help the poor.'

You see, Dad has no interest in money or commerce or material possessions whatsoever. I'm sure he would have much preferred, as a doctor, to never charge his patients anything, which is one reason why he worked so happily in the public hospital system for so many years. I know that many of his patients absolutely revered him, partly because he was such a good doctor, and partly because they could sense that unlike quite a few medical specialists, money was the very last thing he cared about.

He drives around in the most battered old car imaginable, and is completely hopeless when it comes to any sort of mundane, practical domestic matter. He's never changed a light bulb in his life, hammered a nail, mowed a lawn or turned on a washing machine. We used to worry whenever Mum had to go away for any reason, leaving him alone in the house, that he'd starve to death, either because he'd forget to eat, or wouldn't be able to work out how to turn on the oven. He probably wasn't quite as hopeless as he pretended, though. I know he can definitely make a cup of coffee and I have seen him pour milk on a bowl of cereal, so he can manage without Mum, up to a point, though I wouldn't like to see him trying to operate an iron.

Dad displayed the most remarkable courage imaginable during his brain tumour episode. I think this was partly because he just refused to respond the way most ordinary mortals would to that sort of situation.

A day or so after the lengthy operation to remove the tumour, I went to visit him in hospital. I was dreading it, expecting to find him flat on his back, semi-conscious, in great pain, with tubes and drips and monitors all over the place. When I walked in, I found him standing up beside his hospital bed, his head swathed in bandages, doing a cryptic crossword! He explained he was more comfortable standing up. He had 12 fractures in his spine and it was extremely painful to lie on an exceedingly hard hospital mattress, and the staff was far too busy with people dying to worry much about some fellow telling them he had a painful back. As for the crossword, on reflection, he was trying to check, in quite a detached, almost scientific way, if his brain was still functioning.

When we brought him home from hospital, we were assuming he'd sit in the sunroom with a blanket over his legs, and stay that way for several weeks. Certainly, that's what Mum thought he should be doing. He asked me to drive him down the hill to Dee Why beach and drop him there so he could walk up the hill for exercise. Again, I think he just wanted to check how things were functioning, and if he'd sustained any brain damage during the operation. It must have taken almost superhuman willpower for him to walk up the hill that day but he's incredibly stubborn and single-minded. He just decides he's going to do something, regardless of any practical reasons why he shouldn't or can't, and then does it.

Within a very short space of time, only about a month or so, he was insisting on going back to work, despite my mother's howls of protest and despite the fact that he had to undergo a lengthy course of radiotherapy. I used to drive him to his early morning radiotherapy appointment, then drive him across Sydney to Concord Hospital to go to work. I will never forget watching him from the car as he staggered off to the rheumatology department, his body bloated from the massive dose of cortisone he was on to combat the swelling in his brain, his hair all shaven off after the operation, looking absolutely terrible. I couldn't believe anyone could or would do it. But he did!

Within a very short space of time, he was back travelling, and writing articles for medical journals and giving lectures, and jogging and swimming to keep fit.

At the age of 75, he's still travelling around the world and still immersed in sports medicine issues, particularly drugs in sport.

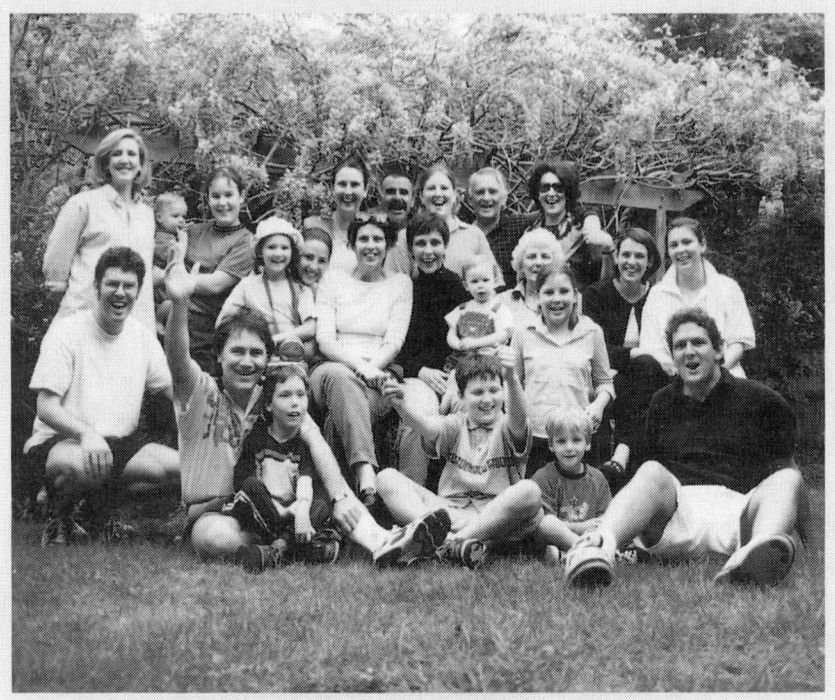

My wonderful family gathered together in 2002 at the golden wedding anniversary of my marriage to Monica. (BRIAN CORRIGAN'S COLLECTION)

Dad has had an amazingly fortunate and privileged life, which I think he'd readily acknowledge, although he's seriously hated growing old and gets very frustrated about it. He and Mum, who two years ago (2002) celebrated their golden wedding anniversary, are never happier than when they are surrounded by family — their five kids, various sons- and daughters-in-law and 14 grandchildren. When we all gather, back at Dee Why, it's quite a crowd! We are all still very close and will always be there for each other.

That's Dad's legacy for the Corrigan family.

'Post-mortem examination revealed that, while she had both male and female chromosomes, the gold medal winner in the Olympic women's 100 metres only had male sex organs. The "she" had always been a "he".'

35. SEX AT THE OLYMPICS

NOW THAT I have your undivided attention, I'm afraid I'm going to disappoint you. This is not really about sex, but rather sex testing at the Olympics.

I do not have any first-hand information about any sex at the Games, none that I can remember anyway, except for one famous romance that was an Olympic version of *West Side Story*. In 1956, the year the Soviet Union invaded Hungary and had the US leaders beating their breasts in outrage, the American gold-medal winning hammer thrower, Harold Connolly, paired off with the Czech gold medal-winning discus thrower, Olga Fikotova, a former basketball champ who practised throwing the discus to the tune of Johann Strauss' *Blue Danube Waltz*. The romance blossomed, much to the consternation of officials from both sides of the Iron Curtain in those Cold War days, but love invariably found its way for they were married in Prague and set up home in California. And lived happily ever after? No, they were divorced in 1973.

THE ANCIENT OLYMPICS, held at Olympia in Greece from 776 BC, lasted for nearly a thousand years, before they were finally ruined following allegations of drug-taking and political interference. Sound familiar? Women were barred from competing under pain of death. Men had to participate in the nude to prove their credentials. However, women *were* allowed to participate in their own Hearea Games, named after Hera, the Goddess of all Gods, at Olympia during the same year as the Olympics.

The Modern Olympics were the brainchild of the nineteenth century Frenchman, Baron Pierre de Coubertin who, with his handpicked royal and military friends, tried to reconstruct their idea of those halcyon days. He was impressed by the English Public School tradition of sportsmanship and muscular Christianity. Throughout his life, he was determinedly opposed to the inclusion of any female competitors, for he thought they were too weak. In the first Modern Olympics held in Athens in 1896, all female competitors were barred.

At Paris in 1900, some female events were on the agenda, including golf and tennis. The women's tennis singles was won by a three-time Wimbledon winner Charlotte Cooper of Great Britain. She went into the history books as the first female Olympic gold medal winner (and she later added another two Wimbledon crowns to her record).

Women have competed in all the Games since then, although few in numbers at first. At Stockholm in 1912, there were 57 female competitors. Women's swimming was included for the first time with the first swimming gold going to Australia when Fanny Durack won the 100-metres freestyle from fellow Aussie Mina Wylie.

After World War I, the Baron's patriarchal attitude and strong opposition to women's participation was shared by his successor, Count Henri de Baillet-Latour. At Amsterdam in 1928, women were permitted to run on the track for the first time in the 100 metres and 800 metres. Several runners collapsed at the finish of the latter race. The Count and many so-called experts seized on this to declare this 'endurance event' too dangerous for females. London's *Daily Mail* newspaper quoted unnamed doctors saying women who ran in the 800 metres would 'become old too soon'. De Baillet-Latour had his way and it was to be 32 years before the race was reinstated, at the 1960 Rome Olympics.

At the 1984 Los Angeles Olympics, the 3000 metres (famous for the fall involving Mary Decker and Zola Budd) and the marathon were first run by woman athletes. The marathon winner was American Joan Benoit, whose time then would have exceeded all the men's gold medal times before 1956.

In 1936, only four sports were available to women — swimming, fencing, athletics and gymnastics. In 1948, the great Dutch runner, Fanny

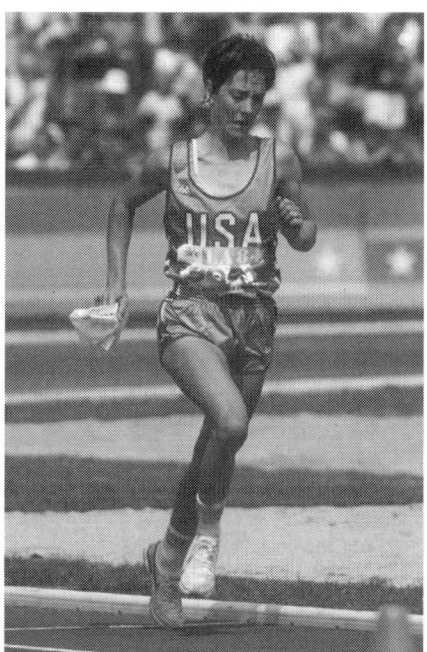 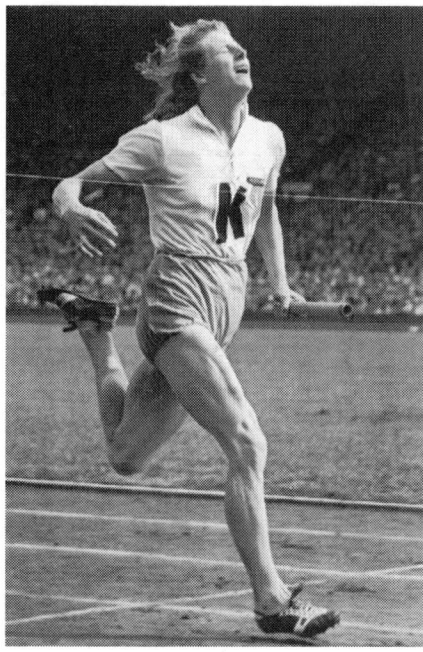

(LEFT) **American Joan Benoit, the gold-medal winner of the first women's Olympic marathon, run at the 1984 Los Angeles Olympics.** (AAP IMAGE/SPORT THE LIBRARY/PRESSE SPORTS). **Fanny Blankers-Koen won three individual gold medals at the 1948 London Olympics, and then won a fourth as a member of the Dutch relay team.** (AAP IMAGE/AP)

Blankers-Koen, won the 100 metres, the new 200 metres, the 80 metres hurdles and was a member of the winning 4 x 100-metres relay team to become the first mother to win gold medals (between her previous appearance, as an 18-year-old at Berlin in 1936, she had married her coach Jan Blankers and given birth to two children). The rules only allowed her to compete in three individual events, so she had to forego both the high jump and the long jump, even though she held the world record in both of these.

Another first occurred in 1956 at the Winter Olympics in Cortina d'Ampezzo, when a female skier, Giuliana Chenal-Minuzzo, took the Olympic oath. Since World War II, the number of women's events at the Summer Olympics has steadily increased, to 23 events in 1992 and 1996, then 25 in Sydney. Similarly, the number of female competitors increased: 610 competitors at Barcelona in 1992, while at Atlanta in 1996 some 3800 women competed, a record up until then. As if to prove that size really does matter, of the 10,300 competitors in Sydney 2000, approximately 40 per cent were women. The noise you could hear was the Baron turning over in his grave.

FOR DECADES, THERE was a widespread conviction among sportswomen that their greatest problem was the possibility of men masquerading as women. Men, with their natural muscular advantage, could compete unfairly by deliberately disguising themselves as women. At almost every Olympics the rumours were rife.

Some women became convinced that the first black female tennis player champion, Althea Gibson, winner of the 1957 and 1958 Wimbledon and US Championships, was a male. Gibson, toughened by a hard life of poverty, was tall, strong and ruthless. Fellow (not intended as a pun) players contrived ways and means to peep at her in the shower to see if they could identify the offending weapon. The hurtful rumours were completely wrong.

Another to suffer the slur was American Mildred 'Babe' Didrikson, arguably the greatest all-round female competitor of all time. She was a champion in all the sports she took up. At the 1932 Los Angeles Olympics she won gold in the 80-metre hurdles (in a world record 11.7 seconds) and javelin (with an Olympic record throw of 43.68 metres) and a silver in the high jump. In the high jump both she and fellow American Jean Shiley cleared a world record height of 1.657 metres, but the judges reckoned Babe's new 'western roll' was illegal because her head cleared the bar before her body and gave the gold to Shirley. A couple of weeks later the authorities legalised the western roll, too late for Babe. The all-round star had actually qualified for five female events, but like Fanny Blankers-Koen was only allowed to compete in three. Babe's brash 'I'm going to beat everybody' image made her many enemies in track and field. She turned to professional golf and became the greatest female player of her era, at one stage winning 14 consecutive tournaments and becoming the first American to win the British Amateur Championship. The other female golfers accused 'Babe' of being a male until the day she died from cancer in September 1956, at the early age of 42. A post-mortem proved, all too late, that the rumours were completely unfounded.

There have been some celebrated (if that is the word) cases of masquerading. Stanislawa Walasiewicz was an expatriate Polish runner, living in the United States under the name of Stella Walsh. At the 1932 Los Angeles she competed for the country of her birth and won the 100-metre sprint, equalling the world record of 11.9 seconds. She had originally wanted to compete for the United States, but had lost her job in the Depression and was saved by an offer of employment from the Polish Consul in New York. Stanislawa ran again in the 1936 Olympics in Berlin, but was beaten into second place by the American sprinter, Helen Stephens, who later claimed that Hitler fondled her bottom while trying to chat her up, finally suggesting a romantic night together at his retreat in Berchtesgaden. He may possibly have gone soft on that idea after the Polish team lodged an official protest at her gold medal success, declaring Stephens to be male. Helen was hauled up before a medical team and suffered the great indignity of having to parade before them naked, before being finally being passed as undoubtedly female.

The Polish protest had simply been a try-on. But there is another twist to this story. Some 44 years later in December 1980, Stella/Stanislawa was shot dead, as seems to happen so many times in America, in a parking lot outside a Cleveland store, as thieves were trying to make their getaway after an armed hold-up. Post-mortem examination revealed that the gold medal winner in the Olympic women's 100 metres only had male sex organs. The 'she' had always been a 'he'.

In 1936, a German high jumper, Dora Ratjen, finished fourth, with a leap of just 2 centimetres less than the gold medal winner, Ibolya Csak of Hungary. Twenty-one years later, Dora confessed that she was really Herman Ratjen. His (or her) story was that he was forced to masquerade as a woman by officials of the Nazi Youth Movement.

One lady in Australia, Mrs Tame, masqueraded as a male throughout his/her life. It may not have mattered much, until he played as a female bowler, entered a lawn bowls championship and won it. The well-hidden secret suddenly became public, and the media had a field day with the story, including the headline, 'No Game for Mrs Tame'.

Things can become a bit more confused when you consider that some females have a natural male appearance, but are unquestionably female. This could apply to some of today's female athletes and tennis players, especially since the introduction of weight training.

Alternatively, women who take anabolic steroids become remarkably male-like in appearance. Recent examples of this have been some of the Chinese swimmers who were on steroids. The outspoken Aussie swim coach Laurie Laurence reckoned they had shoulders that would have done a world champion axeman proud. Everyone will also remember the massive build of the East German women swimmers and athletes in the 1970s, compared with athletes such as the Australian sprinter Raelene Boyle who had to compete against them. Some of the East Germans would have done well playing in the second row of the Australian Rugby League Test team. Raelene, who was a hell of a lot of woman, but sometimes not very lady-like, said after finishing second behind one of them: 'That's the first time I have been beaten by someone with balls.'

The World Veterans' Athletic Championship held at the northern English town of Gateshead in 1999 produced a great controversy. Everyone was amazed at the muscular build of the American world champion runner, 56-year-old Kathy Jager. So much so that the Australian and New Zealand teams laid an official complaint, suggesting she was a male masquerading as a woman.

'I told them that would be a real surprise to my husband, two children and four grandchildren,' Jager suggested. After testing, she was shown to be female, but she was found guilty of taking anabolic steroids, which were apparently part of a hormone replacement therapy for her change of life.

TRANSSEXUALS ARE PEOPLE who have a deep, ineradicable belief they have been born the wrong gender. When gender reassignment, better known as a sex change operation, became available, some former athletes, including some champions, underwent this surgery.

Here are some examples.

Austrian Erika Schineggar won the women's world downhill skiing championship in 1966. She retired the following year, became a man, then returned as Erik, competed once again at top level and also later became a father.

An American ophthalmologist and better than average tennis player, Richard Raskin, had a sex change and became Renee Richards. In 1976, at the age of 42, Renee attempted to compete in women's events, much to the anguish of the other players who wanted her banned. She took the US tennis authorities to court, forcing them to allow her to play. The ruling was regarded as an important precedent for all sports.

An Australian male runner, Ricki Carne, underwent this long and difficult operation and in 1991 competed in female events and won several races. Although Ricki was of only moderate ability, female officialdom threw a willy (so to speak) and did everything possible to prevent her running. Their efforts were thwarted when Athletics Australia ruled that there was no provision for gender identification for domestic events. The Carne case was even debated in the State Parliament of New South Wales.

A similar problem was reported in 1995 when a golf player, Lana (previously Alan) Barlow, wrote to her South Australian golf club after a sex change operation requesting to be allowed to play now as a woman. Women's Golf Australia agreed to it, but there were still problems with other competitors. Lana later lent her support to another golfer, 32-year-old Mianne Bagger, who was born a male. Bagger won the 1999 South Australian Amateur Championship with the full blessing of the golf authorities.

IT MAY BE hard to believe, but let me assure you it is true, that it can be difficult at times to distinguish males from females. In order for the human foetus to develop into either a male or female, all the biological systems responsible must be on 'Go'. If something is not quite right with the 'Go' switch, a whole range of medical conditions encompassing people who appear outwardly male but are internally female, to those who appear female but are males, can occur. Sometimes it can take a great deal of investigation to make certain what the true gender is. Hermaphrodites, for example, have both male and female attributes equally. All these changes are known collectively as the problem of intersex.

Consider for a moment how these changes could more easily be detected among female sporting athletes. The first method, one to which women athletes naturally objected strenuously, required them to parade in the nude before a medical panel. Things became worse in Jamaica in 1966, when, at what was then called the British Empire and Commonwealth Games, some athletes had to submit to a gynaecological examination. Complaints about this treatment finally forced the IOC to act, and athletes were saved, not by the bell, but by the Barr body test. Which brings us to the subject of sex testing, or to give it its official title, gender verification.

THE NUCLEUS OF female body cells contains two X chromosomes, and the two chromosomes together are readily detected under the microscope as a distinct dark-coloured body, named a Barr body after the scientist who discovered it (Dr Murray Barr). On the other hand, the male nucleus has two chromosomes, but they are different. One is still called X but the other is Y. The single X chromosome in males does not show up in the Barr body test.

This sex chromatin test is easy to perform, all that is required are a few body cells, easily obtained by smearing the inside of the mouth or pulling out a hair. I remember the first time we performed the test in Sydney, before the Mexico Olympics in 1968. All female competitors turned up, accompanied by anxious looking mothers. Invariably Mum's first question would be, 'How is this test going to be performed?' On telling them a swab was taken from the mouth, Mum would visibly relax and interrupt to say, 'From her mouth?' and then to her daughter, 'Oh, that's all right then, love.' The only person who was exempted from having the test was Princess Anne, when she competed in her equestrian event.

It seemed like a marvellous test in those very early days. Feminine dignity was preserved and the sport scientists would have a simple test that would also detect the problems of men masquerading as women and doubts about intersex.

Some previously suspect athletes simply disappeared from the scene, retiring, or so it was announced. The Soviet Union had two stars who between them had won five Olympic gold medals and set 26 world records, Iryna and Tamara Press. Iryna had won the 80-metre hurdles at the 1960 Rome Olympics and the inaugural pentathlon in Tokyo four years later. Tamara won gold in the shot-put at both Rome and Tokyo and a silver (1960) and gold (1964) in the discus. The pair was better known to us as the Press brothers. After sex tests were introduced they were never seen again, ever.

In 1967, it seemed the scientists had, like the Canadian Mounties, finally got their man, as the first test with an abnormal result was found. Polish sprinter Eva Klobukowska, a world and Olympic champion was tested at the European Championships in Kiev and was found to have a relatively common intersex disorder. She had an extra X chromosome with internal male testes. She probably had no idea that there was any sort of problem before it was announced that she had failed the test.

Many of us noted the terrible humiliation, injustice and psychic trauma for the poor girl in being made an example of before the rest of the world.

IT DID NOT take very long at all before a scientific fly was found in the IOC's ointment. Medical opinion considered the Barr body test to be technically unreliable and not completely foolproof. Not long afterwards virtually all laboratories gradually began to abandon the test. It really had been too simplistic to think that such a test could or would accurately sort out the many potentially complex problems of sex identification. Many bodily changes can be attributed to intersex, and many variations are possible within the X and Y chromosomes. Moreover, some of the genetic changes that the test revealed did not confer any athletic advantage at all.

Many experts also disagreed with the test on ethical grounds. They argued that tests of this nature should be confined to the privacy of a medical consultation room, and that fully informed consent to perform them should be compulsory. No such protection could be offered to an athlete under the hothouse conditions of Olympic sex testing. It was a human tragedy of the highest order, capable of causing irreparable psychological damage, to label someone as being a male when up until then they had always been regarded as being a female, all as the result of such an unreliable test. Once the test result was announced, there was usually little the athlete in question could do.

Not so for Maria Patino, a Spanish hurdler who, because of an underlying genetic problem, failed this test at the 1985 World Student Games in Kobe, Japan, and was labelled male. Her team bosses advised her to fake an injury and leave the Games. She was so incensed with this suggestion that she decided not to go quietly. It took Patino two and a half years, but she ultimately won and the International Amateur Athletics Federation (IAAF) backed down and agreed she was a woman after all.

All this controversy wasn't seen to be a problem by the IOC, who continued to use the Barr body as the main test for female Olympic athletes until 2000. Some modifications were made and tests were improved, but no advancements in technology could really answer the major problems and criticisms of the flawed test.

If you wonder why this test was continued for so long after it had been discredited, it was the women athletes who kept pushing to keep it. There was some justification for the IOC; for women did not want to lose what for them was such a simple test to perform, and they feared that any change would be for the worse. At the Brisbane Commonwealth Games in 1982, the women's lawn bowling team, all grandmothers, turned up for gender verification. When told they really did not need to take the test, as having had a child was definite proof of femininity, they were incensed, alleged they were being discriminated against and demanded to be tested. In the end, it became easier to perform the test than to argue with them, but the media really gave us heaps for testing the poor old grannies.

In 1996, female Olympic athletes were asked two questions concerning whether or not this form of testing should be continued. Of the 928 who responded, 82 per cent said it should be continued, with 94 per cent saying that they were happy with the procedure and found it reassuring.

In the end, though, so many protests were flooding in to the IOC about this test — not only from scientific groups but also from sporting groups such as the IAAF, and also some female athletic groups — that the IOC was forced to act. It was also running the risk of being sued for unfair discrimination against those women with gender abnormalities who received no advantage as far as athletic prowess was concerned. By the time the Sydney Games arrived, it was decided that, since so little was to be gained by continuing the Barr body test, it would be much better to abandon it as the form of sex testing altogether. It seemed likely that the major problem of masquerading was no longer such a problem, as everyone had to agree to a supervised urine drug test, where all would be revealed.

The IOC may also have been thinking that, with the skimpiness of sports gear worn nowadays, it would be impossible for any male to masquerade as a female anyway. In 2004, the Committee also allowed transexuals to complete.

'We have seen schoolchildren of 12 or 10 given steroids, usually by their parents or sports coach.'

36. PANDORA'S BOX

BY FAR THE greatest problem facing the Olympic Movement is undoubtedly that of drugs in sport. They are banned for two very good reasons. One is the harm done as a result of their side effects. The second is that taking performance-enhancing drugs is a form of cheating, deliberate cheating, and contrary to the spirit and purpose of fair competition. If you don't believe it is cheating, I would ask you to talk to any of those athletes or swimmers who finished second behind the East German juggernauts in the 1980s, or more recently the Chinese steroid-built swimmers. The East Germans and Chinese robbed genuine sportsmen and women of gold medals. Sport was surely never intended to be a competition between guinea pigs who are being doped by various pharmaceutical agents.

Sportspeople, as with the rest of the community, may need to use many different types of medications for a legitimate medical reason. This includes antibiotics, treatments for most stomach disorders, and anti-inflammatory agents, which are permitted in humans, but banned in horse racing, because they can mask an injury, and a hard-driven horse can easily snap a tendon or bone. This happened in late 2002 in Western Australia when a horse ridden by jockey Jason Oliver fell and both jockey and horse died. These medications are not what we are talking about here.

People have been searching for some magical substance to enhance the performance of mind and body for millennia. One example is the

'Alice in Wonderland Syndrome' taking its name from when Alice found a cake marked 'Eat Me', which she did and became larger. Users of anabolic steroids are still firm believers in this fairytale.

I've already mentioned how one of the major reasons for the break-up of the original Olympic Games some 2000 years ago was the abuse of drugs. The drugs used then, such as the rear hooves of an ass served up with rose petals, may now seem to be harmless concoctions. But some, such as herbs, mushrooms and hallucinogens, may have been particularly dangerous. The Scandinavian Berserkers used mushrooms to send themselves 'berserk' before terrorising their neighbours and anyone else who happened to get in their way. One popular 'tonic' before the turn of the nineteenth century, Vin Mariani, contained cocaine and was favoured by Popes Pius X and Leo XIII, and, dare I say it, Queen Victoria.

The 'win at any cost' mentality that has caused such harm in sport began in the nineteenth century when the common agents used included the poisons strychnine and nitro-glycerine. Cyclists, then as now, were frequent drug users and in 1886 a Welsh cyclist Arthur Linton died after taking a stimulant during the famous Paris–Bordeaux race. It is the first reported death of a sportsman from doping.

The word 'dope' derives from 'dop', a strong liquor popular with South African natives. The word was derived from the Dutch word *doop*, a thick sauce that people dipped into. About 1890, thick preparations of opium also came to be called dope. Doping was then applied to similar types of drugs, especially a drug to influence horse races or impair a performance. In 1910 when the world boxing champion, Jack Johnson, lost his title, he claimed he had been doped.

In the Olympics, the first near death occurred in the marathon at St Louis in 1904. Some 16 kilometres from the finish the American, Thomas Hicks, who was leading wanted to pull out. His handlers would hear nothing of it and for the remainder of the race kept giving him doses of a mixture of brandy and strychnine. In a stupor, Hicks won the race by 6 minutes but collapsed over the finishing line and never ran again. The first death occurred in the marathon at the 1912 Stockholm Games when the 21-year-old Portuguese runner, Francisco Lazaro, collapsed in the heat and died next day in hospital.

The second Olympic death, that of Danish cyclist Kurt Jensen in the Team Time Trial at Rome in 1960 was particularly sad and unnecessary since he took a combination of amphetamines and a drug to dilate the blood vessels, taken in the mistaken belief they would increase blood flow through his muscles. This did not work and in the 35 degree heat of Rome he collapsed and died. Two other Danes also collapsed and had to be hospitalised after taking drugs.

In the following years, deaths in sport continued as virtually any substance athletes believed might improve performance were used, often in very high dosages. Most problems occurred with amphetamines, the most well-known incident being that of Tommy Simpson, the champion English cyclist, who died during the 1967 Tour de France while climbing the 1850 metre Mont Ventouse after taking amphetamines.

As other cases became known, the semantic wrangling about the definition of drugs that had been going on for many years had to end. Accordingly, in 1967, before the Mexico Olympics, the IOC produced their first definition of doping, and the Olympic chiefs published a list of banned substances, which were not to be taken under *any* circumstances.

Most, but not quite all, sporting organisations adopted this IOC list, although there were problems, especially with uniform interpretation in different countries and different sports. The task of sorting all this out and ensuring uniformity has fallen to the World Anti-Drug Agency (WADA), under the chairmanship of the Canadian lawyer and IOC member, Dick Pound. Features of the first ever global anti-doping code include: a single list of prohibited substances, uniform drug testing regulations and sanctions for all sports and countries, plus a ban on *genetic doping*. This code will supersede the IOC list and sport associations are required to enact it by the 2004 Athens Olympics.

THE FIRST LIST of banned substances supplied by the IOC contained stimulants and depressants, but was subsequently increased to include the following substances, which should show the extremes and risks some athletes will take to win.

Amphetamines, more commonly known as speed, were first used by American troops and pilots to keep themselves awake during World War II and later became common throughout the sporting world. During the 1960s and 1970s, their use was particularly widespread. As one coach said, he handed out different coloured ones like lollies. Amphetamines increase mental alertness and aggression, with the very small side-effect of improving performance. They are still used to this day, although not nearly so commonly as in the 1960s.

Next on the list are anabolic steroids. Testosterone, the male sex hormone produced in the testes — the 'gland of hope and glory' my University tutor used to call it — is an anabolic steroid. Anabolic means to build up and steroids are a common body constituent, for example, cholesterol is a steroid. Testosterone was used by the Germans during World War II for its ability to enhance aggressiveness. Soviet athletes in Helsinki 1952 were suspected, and it was subsequently verified, to be using testosterone to increase muscle strength and power. The Americans, quick to find alternatives to testosterone, developed similar compounds, the anabolic steroids. These became generally available in 1958, and Pandora's Box of sporting drugs was opened.

At first, sports scientists made one colossal blunder. After researching the scientific literature, they stated that anabolic steroids did not have any beneficial effects on muscle performance, but the research was based on only small doses of steroid. Administering huge doses was unethical, so proper scientific trials were never conducted. The cheating athletes were taking massive doses. The IOC eventually realised the athletes were laughing at them as the sports stars' muscle bulk increased and world records fell. Anabolic steroids were finally added to the IOC's banned list in 1974, even though no really reliable test for them was available at that time. And the athletes knew it.

Because so many different types of steroids were at this time available, the words 'and related substances' were added to the list. During the 1980s, the East Germans employed doctors to manage their athletes' use of anabolic steroids with devastating effects on the athletes' health.

The problem with anabolic steroids has shifted from their widespread use by elite athletes to their current use by body builders, nightclub bouncers and others who may have no real interest in sport but who want to impress with their physique. Even worse, their use has spread to teenagers and even young children. We have seen schoolchildren of ten or twelve years of age given steroids, usually by their parents or sports coach.

Perhaps, worst of all, is their use by women, often given to them by their bodybuilding boyfriends. Females suffer even greater side effects than males.

Since the 1980s, the IOC's list of prohibited drugs has grown like a weed. Since 1985 it has included:

Diuretics are water loss tablets that will always be associated, in Australia at least, with cricketer Shane Warne. He said he took them to control his weight and was given them by his mother. Any reduction in weight is, of course, due to water loss, not fat, and will be replaced with the first glass of water. Diuretics are used medically to treat high blood pressure and heart failure when excessive body fluid accumulates. They are also used by sportspeople, such as wrestlers, weightlifters or jockeys, who need to make the 'correct' weight for their event. In such cases, the drugs are often used in very high doses. This can be particularly dangerous to their health as essential minerals are lost. The other use for diuretics is by steroid abusers in the mistaken belief that, by diluting the urine, steroids will not be detected. This is no problem for the laboratory. Modern tests simply detect the presence of the diuretic plus the original steroid.

It may seem strange to have alcohol on the list, especially since it is much more usual to consume it after an event than before it. Shooters and Modern Pentathlon competitors had used it for years. Pentathaletes said, and could prove, that their performances in four of their events were always slightly better during competition than in training. The other event, shooting, was always slightly worse in competition due to increased sharpness of reflexes. Alcohol was taken to dampen down the unwanted reactions in the shooting regime and a certain blood alcohol level was permitted. It is claimed that the authorities changed their minds about allowing alcohol to be consumed when one shooter — he had to be Irish, didn't he? — had a few too many and some of his shots went perilously close to the officials. But by then beta-blockers, much more efficient and easier to manage, had become readily available.

Beta-blockers are commonly used in medicine to decrease anxiety, reduce hand tremors and slow the heart rate. They can also be used by shooters for the same reasons. A slower heart rate can also be very useful because shooters can train themselves to time their shots between heartbeats. And reducing the slight, normally present minute hand tremor enables them to shoot more accurately.

It may also seem strange to ban caffeine, a universal stimulant in everyday use. It is present in coffee, tea, chocolate … and sportspeople. It must be remembered that it is an 'upper' that increases the heart rate and alertness and overcomes tiredness. It can be taken in very high doses by using tablets or injections. Some athletes have been known to eat Nescafé by the spoonful. Caffeine was placed on the banned list in 1983. Some allowance had to be made because of its everyday use, so a certain amount of caffeine was allowed to be present in the urine tests. There was a level of 12 units, above this a test would be considered positive. In the Seoul Olympic Games in 1988, there were 1600 urine tests performed for caffeine and all in the range of two to three units, well below the cut-off level of 12. One Australian competitor in the Modern Pentathlon, Alex Watson, had a level of 14.1, a result that stood out like a sore thumb. He was considered positive, the IOC banned him for two years, and the Australian Olympic Federation (AOF) for life (later reducing the penalty to a two-year disqualification). A Senate inquiry later showed that, while the level of caffeine was definitely too high, there was no evidence that Watson had been responsible for the levels. The AOF was accused of over-reacting.

Alex may have been a trifle unlucky. Subsequently, research showed that there were so many problems with, and doubts about, test levels that WADA decided testing for caffeine should be discontinued.

From the everyday to the more extreme tampering tricks:

First up, blood doping. This is a technique where some of one's own blood is removed and stored. The body quickly makes up the deficiency. The stored blood can be returned to the body later to boost blood levels just before performing. This had been suspected since 1972, when Scandinavians perfected the technique. It was rumoured that Finnish long-distance star Lasse Viren, who won the 5000 metres and 10,000 metres at the Munich Olympics in 1972, and then won both events again four years later, was using it.

The Scandinavians categorically denied using blood doping, but at the Los Angeles Olympics in 1984, another Finnish distance runner, Marti Vainio, tested positive for steroids. He denied taking them, well, not for six months anyway. He had stored some blood with which to 'blood dope' himself at the Games, and the re-introduced blood contained the steroids he had taken months earlier. Very unlucky.

In 1984, several members of the American cycling team did admit to their involvement in blood doping at a Los Angeles hotel room. Some of them became mighty ill and could not complete their commitments at the Games.

Besides the risk of infections, transfusions are known to cause severe reactions. The IOC banned blood doping in 1986, even though there was no method of detecting it.

EPO is a powerful bone marrow booster that increases the body's production of blood cells. EPO was first used medically in 1985 for the successful treatment of severe anaemia. Athletes took up its use enthusiastically, for it meant there would no longer be any need for the cumbersome blood doping methods. EPO abuse is now common. In 1998 an entire cycling team was dismissed from the Tour de France for using it.

Medical complications soon became evident because EPO causes the blood to thicken, forming a sludge and makes it difficult for blood to pass through the smaller blood vessels. Complications including heart attacks, stroke and death in cyclists have been reported.

In 1990, EPO was added to the banned list, but continued to be a problem because it remained for such a short time in the system that a blood test would seemingly be necessary for its detection and no such test was available then. Just before the Sydney Olympics in 2000 a combined blood and urine test became available. Since then the urine test has been modified and had become more acceptable.

Human growth hormone has also been added to the list. Its legitimate use was to help stunted children to grow. Athletes latched on to the growth hormone because of its muscle-building properties, but since most other body tissues increase as well, side effects can be disastrous. To date, no effective urine test has become available, but one is said to be imminent and it will be necessary to develop a blood test.

'A caller came to collect a random test one morning, but Michelle Smith's urine mysteriously became contaminated by alcohol.'

37. CATCHING THE CHEATS

AS EXPLAINED, THERE are good reasons why many of the drugs used in sport are prohibited, and why it is essential to have a proper stringent system to detect their presence. In the past, this system has been based only on urine tests, until blood testing was initiated at the 2000 Sydney Olympics.

The first methods used for drug detection were relatively crude. At the beginning of the twentieth century testing relied on identifying colour changes in drug crystals, so a reliable method of testing became a major necessity. Real success came with the introduction of advanced technology during the 1970s. Precise and accurate identification of drugs in the most minute quantities is now possible with an instrument known as a Gas Chromatography Mass Spectrometer (or GC-MS), in which a substance can be identified with what is essentially a chemical fingerprint. This can then be compared against a computer reference library of several thousand compounds.

The tests have until recently been conducted in accordance with a long IOC list of prohibited drugs and their methods of use, updated every year and circulated to all sporting bodies. There are some problems with this list, which for some time has needed an overhaul. One problem is that the various sports have different rules and regulations concerning how the tests are to be handled. Some restrict all drugs on the IOC list, some restrict certain drugs only; some have different penalties, especially regarding the length of time that bans are imposed; some, such as asthma medications, are allowed only after vetting by a medical body. The task of sorting all this out has also fallen to WADA. Urine testing was first carried out at the Mexico Olympics when specimens were required from the first four place-getters in selected events and another two could be chosen at random. The first runner to be tested was Ron Clarke.

Urine is much preferred to blood for drug testing, for several good reasons. It is easer to collect, transport and store than blood, and is much easier to handle in the laboratory. Some people, especially in the media and among retired athletes, believe that blood should always be used and if not, there must be some conspiracy to prevent its use. The truth is that urine is a better medium for detecting all drugs, except for Growth Hormone (for which no test, urine or blood, is available) and EPO, which required both urine and blood tests.

When urine is used, scrupulous care in its collection and labelling is mandatory. The number of tests required at a sporting event varies. In individual events, such as running or swimming, it is usually the first three or four place-getters. In team events, such as cricket or football, usually two or three sportspeople are chosen. The Drug Control Officer meets those selected and stays with them, not letting them out of sight, until they reach the Drug Control Office where the doctor or technical officer who is to perform the test is waiting. Refusal to attend is, of course, regarded as the same as having a positive result.

The athlete remains under constant observation by a same sex drug testing official while urine is collected. This act of deliberate voyeurism is necessary because many tricks have been attempted, such as a rubber tube with clean urine inserted into the bladder or the urine specimen substituted with another clean one, or the specimen may be adulterated. The most famous case of this occurred with the Irish swimmer, Michelle Smith, later Michelle de Bruin, whose swimming times suddenly and dramatically improved at the 1996 Atlanta Olympics. Some time later, a caller came to collect a random test one morning, but Michelle Smith's urine mysteriously became contaminated by alcohol.

The urine sample is then poured into a sealed, sterilised beaker, chosen at random by the athlete. It has to be of a sufficient volume, which can be a problem when it happens that you have to sit around until a very late hour, waiting for the athlete to feel the urge. The office is well stocked with drinks, but no beer or caffeine-containing Coca-Cola.

Two other tests are then carried out. One is to test how acid the urine is, the other how dilute it is. Urine gets more acidic with exercise, especially after heavy or prolonged exercise. If the urine sample is not sufficiently acidic, suspicions would be raised about possible tampering. On the other hand, dilute urine can also indicate attempts at tampering or the taking of diuretics. The athlete is then asked about the medications he or she has taken over the past three days, including all tablets, injections, suppositories, inhalations, ointment and vitamins, minerals and supplements.

The Drug Control Official records all the information on the designated form, which also acts as the record of the chain-of-custody procedures right up to the laboratory. The paperwork is divided, like Caesar's Gaul, into three parts. One page is given to the athlete and one to the sporting authority ordering the test. The main point here is that the third page that goes to the laboratory does not include the athlete's name, only a number, so the laboratory never knows which athlete is being tested, despite some rumours to the contrary. Accurate detailed records of the whole procedure are necessary, for any part may subsequently come under intense legal and scientific scrutiny. One incorrectly crossed 'T' or undotted 'I' may cause a fury from the hovering, scrutinising lawyers, claiming the most minute error as incontrovertible evidence the test has been incorrectly performed.

The urine is divided into two containers, both of which are sealed, numbered and dispatched to the testing laboratory. The laboratory, like Caesar's wife, has to be above suspicion. The IOC-controlled testing laboratories undergo rigorous examination each year and just one small error, even in the interpretation of a test result, can mean deregistration. Fair enough too, for they hold an athlete's reputation and livelihood in their hands.

All samples must also be correctly stored and refrigerated if they are to reflect the body's composition accurately. Urine cannot be left in the sun as this can alter the test with some naturally present steroids converted to illegal steroids. This happened to British runner Diane Modahl, a former winner of the Commonwealth Games 800 metres. Her specimen was left out in the sun one particularly hot day in Lisbon in 1994. Her sample returned a high positive test for steroids and she was suspended for four years. She appealed to an independent body, which found in her favour.

The presence in urine of a banned substance, or traces of its breakdown products, is sufficient to constitute a positive test. In other words, it is not incumbent upon the testing body to determine how that substance got into the body; if it's there, then the test is positive.

One specimen, called A, is tested first, while the second, B, is kept in reserve for a repeat analysis should it be needed. If the A sample tests negative, the urine can be discarded. If it is positive, the athlete has the right to have the reserve sample tested in front of witnesses of their choice. This does seem like an act of desperation, in the hope — invariably a vain hope — that the B sample might produce a different result. But retesting it is the athlete's prerogative.

Technology has made a huge difference in drug detection. The modern testing machine, the GC-MS, is compulsory in all IOC-controlled laboratories and is as close to foolproof as it's possible to get. Which brings us to two common problems associated with drug testing, therapeutic and inadvertent use of banned substances.

THERAPEUTIC USE IS very much in the news these days, as athletes may need to use a drug on the IOC list of banned substances for legitimate treatment of a medical condition. That the therapeutic use of drugs for athletes should be penalised is obviously unjust and unnecessary, and in many instances beyond common sense. Medical advisory panels have been set up in some countries and also by some international bodies to collect and assess the evidence concerning the need for the therapeutic use of these types of problems and advise accordingly, a welcome development.

Here are a few examples of the type of problem encountered.

Steroids are a case in point. One cause of confusion is the word steroid, as the body contains many naturally occurring steroids. Cholesterol, for example, is one naturally occurring steroid, as is cortisone and the male and female sex hormones. Some of these natural steroids are used for therapeutic purposes. Cortisone, for example, is prescribed for a variety of medical conditions, including arthritis or other forms of inflammation. The problem arises as some athletes use cortisone in very high doses for very dubious reasons. Anabolic steroids, however, are a different problem — they are not naturally occurring, have to be administered from outside the body, and medical reasons for their use are quite rare.

ADD, or more recently ADHD, Attention Deficit Hyperactivity Disorder, was considered to be a particularly uncommon problem involving small children who would grow out of it by the age of 16. It has since been found to be quite a common problem, which children rarely grow out of and which can occur in much older people. Different strategies are needed, but the most common treatment is with stimulants, usually given as Ritalin, which is related to amphetamines. These drugs have a paradoxical effect in that hyperactive children become much calmer and more manageable.

The banned masking agents, Benemid and diuretics, receive a fair share of media coverage. Anabolic steroid users use them in an attempt to mask drug use. Benemid is also used to treat gout, although its use as a treatment for gout has been largely superseded. Of more importance, Benemid is also given to people on penicillin treatment because it increases the amount of penicillin in the blood. There have been recent cases of athletes who needed high doses of penicillin and were unknowingly given Benemid by their doctors, and testing positive for this banned substance.

Asthma presents another similar problem. The commonly used puffers contain Ventolin, which is also on the IOC banned list. The puffers contain only relatively low doses of Ventolin and there are no problems with this dose. Ventolin can also be taken in high doses, usually by tablets, when it is also anabolic. Nevertheless, there has been so much confusion and problems with the testing of Ventolin that WADA will cease testing for it.

INADVERTENT USE IS the accidental or unknowing use of a banned substance contained in a commonly available medication and is a different problem. In practice, this usually comes down to products sold over-the-counter for coughs or colds. The substance they contain is usually some form of the stimulant ephedrine, which is itself closely related to, or derived from, amphetamine.

We are not speaking here of a teaspoon dose of a decongestant every now and again. Rather, athletes may take up to a third of a bottle at a time. The problem with such doses is that the side effects of ephedrine can be horrendous and include sudden death and strokes.

It would seem to be a bit unrealistic to expect doctors to consult the list of IOC banned drugs every time a patient who happens to be an athlete comes in. There is now a much greater awareness of the problem in sports and athletes are constantly being warned of the risks involved, and sport organisations have trained people available to give proper advice.

All sportspeople are warned repeatedly never to take any form of medication without first checking with appropriate authorities.

'Most supplements, with few exceptions, have never been proved to be of any value in improving performance ...'

38. SYDNEY 2000 DRUG TESTING

THE OLYMPICS HELD in Sydney in September 2000 were attended by 10,300 athletes, 2758 of whom (1616 males and 1141 females — and, yes, you're right, that does not add up because the sex of one was not stated) became available for drug testing.

Urine tests were collected from three separate sites. A total of 2148 were collected during the two weeks of the Games and 437 tests were conducted over a four-week period before the competition for the first time in Olympic history. There were 310 blood tests (another Olympic first) and with these were 315 urine samples (again these figures do not add up correctly, because for technical reasons some urine tests needed to be repeated).

There had been much debate before the Games whether or not blood tests constituted some breach of civil liberties. The answer from the IOC Medical Commission was unequivocal. No athlete is forced to compete, but any who do must obey these rules. Experienced technicians performed the blood tests and no problems or objections were encountered.

All urine and blood tests were analysed at the Australian Drug Testing Laboratory in the Sydney suburb of Pymble, under the direction of Dr Ray Kazlauskas. He and his team of 90 scientists worked around the clock to provide a rapid turn-around time of one to two days for the results.

Throughout the Games, eleven tests returned a positive result for drugs on the banned list. This included five medal winners. They did, of course, lose their medals.

All 2758 tested competitors were asked the same question: 'What medications have you taken in the past three days?' Interpreters were provided for all languages, if required. The answers to that question included the whole range of medications, prescription drugs, over-the-counter medications, those taken by mouth, injected, inhaled, ointments and suppositories, plus all vitamins, minerals, and food supplements. The answers were reviewed and have subsequently been published. The three most commonly abused medications in this survey were vitamins and minerals, asthma preparations; and the non-steroidal anti-inflammatory agents.

The number of medications taken in a day provided some fascinating statistics. Most athletes took only one or two supplements in a day. However, 542 athletes took five or more in a day. The most was one athlete who took 26 separate items in one day, while some took 20, and some 18. You would have to wonder how the money or time to swallow such inordinate amounts could be found. The answer is, of course, they didn't pay for these things themselves, as most were given to them free for promotional purposes. An interesting example was the Australian soccer team, some of whom took vitamin supplements when given free, but none used them at home when they had to pay for them out of their own pockets. The problem is that most supplements, with few exceptions, have never been proved to be of any value in improving performance and may be looked upon as expensive placebos. It was most gratifying to hear from Dr Brian Sando, who was in charge of the Australian swimming team at these Olympics, that the leading Australian male and female swimmers did not see any need to take supplements.

You might think that the athletes who took such large amounts of supplements might be embarrassed or diffident about owning up to taking so many. Not at all! They were so proud of this and insisted that all supplements be recorded. 'Make sure you write them all down' was a common statement.

SECOND OPINION

PROFESSOR KEN FITCH

World-renowned expert on drugs in sport. Attached to the University of Western Australia's school of human movement and exercise science, Ken is the Australian Sports Drug Agency's chief medical advisor and a member of the International Olympic Committee's medical commission. He was appointed to oversee all sports medicine services at the 2000 Sydney Olympics.

INSTANT RAPPORT

I FIRST MET Alfred Brian Corrigan, or ABC as I call him, when he came to Perth in 1965 for a sports medicine conference. He was the eleventh hour replacement for another expert who had taken ill. That expert had intended staying with my family and me, so I extended the same invitation to ABC even though I had never heard of him and knew nothing about him. We met at Perth Airport and we were firm friends by the time we had driven the 25 minutes to my home. He stayed about a week and fitted into my family (including four children aged between one and seven years) as though he had known us all of his life. For me, that week had a major effect on my life. Brian helped clarify my future. By the time he left I was resolved to obtain more qualifications in sports and physical medicine just as he had done.

Soon after, I became Federal Secretary of the Australian Sports Medicine Federation (now Sports Medicine Australia) and ABC, the Vice-President and then National President. We worked very closely and harmoniously through some difficult and testing times for the fledgling body.

Munich 1972 remains a highlight of our long association. The 1968 Mexico City Games (his first) had not been as enjoyable for ABC as anticipated and he was determined that Munich would be different. Although he was the senior and I was the junior team doctor, from the outset he insisted that we were equal and shared the work and responsibilities. It was a memorable and huge learning experience for me, living in the same flat for six weeks and observing him work.

We were also members of the Australian Olympic medical teams in Moscow 1980 and Los Angeles 1984. Later associations included our involvement in setting up the Australian Sports Drug Agency (ASDA) in Canberra and the Australian Sports Drugs Testing Laboratory (ASDTL) in Sydney and as members of the Medical Advisory Panel of the Australian Sports Commission.

As a doctor, ABC's clinical skills were always exceptional. He had the ability to develop instant rapport with and the confidence of every patient, of both genders and of any age. Taking the patient's history was always unhurried and skilful but his examination of the musculoskeletal system was without doubt the best that I have ever encountered in any other sports health professional. This may have been assisted by enrolling as an 'alleged' physiotherapist in a course conducted by Dr Cyriax, a leader in manipulative medicine, in London during the early 1960s. It may have been further refined by his association with the South Australian father and doyen of manipulative therapy, Geoff Maitland with whom ABC wrote a major textbook.

ABC had another side to him. It was mischievous but never malicious or hateful. In 1979 he invited me to present a keynote lecture on 'Running Injuries' at the Concord Hospital's Annual Post Graduate Week. I left my practice for three or four days, flew over and stayed with the Corrigans in Dee Why. After presenting an hour-long lecture including questions, ABC then asked me for my slides that had taken me several weeks to put together. When asked why, his response was: 'I'm going to England on Saturday and have to present a lecture on the same subject. I asked you to Sydney to save me having to prepare a lecture.' Cheeky devil, it seems I was his unpaid research assistant. Of course, I had no hesitation in helping out my mate.

There was the time in the 1980s when ABC was found to have a brain tumour. Like all of his friends, I was devastated. A few days after he left hospital, I was in Melbourne for a Saturday commitment and organised with his wife Monica to come to Sydney. I had done this on several occasions in the past but always with anticipation of a great day with ABC, however I was anxious about seeing him. I drove him in his car to a spot near a beach south of Dee Why and we spoke with complete openness about many matters. Although his mental capacity had not completely returned to normal, I was pleasantly surprised with his cerebral function but still fearful of his future. To everyone's delight, ABC regained all of his mental faculties — except perhaps one or two that made him an even better bloke! His output of writing since his tumour and his acquisition of computer literacy has been outstanding.

For many years, we used to communicate by mail. My letters were almost illegible; his were abbreviated notes written suddenly on any piece of paper that he could lay his hands on when the need to write became imperative. Since we have both began using computers, he is delighted that my communications are legible and I am pleased that his appear on a computer screen instead of any old piece of paper!

Despite his many and often long absences from Monica and their four daughters and son, often at important periods of the children's lives and development, all his children are devoted to their father. He is so important to them. Monica has always been there for Brian and the family.

Even though we have lived on opposite sides of Australia, ABC has been one of my closest colleagues and most respected and dear friends for nearly 40 years.

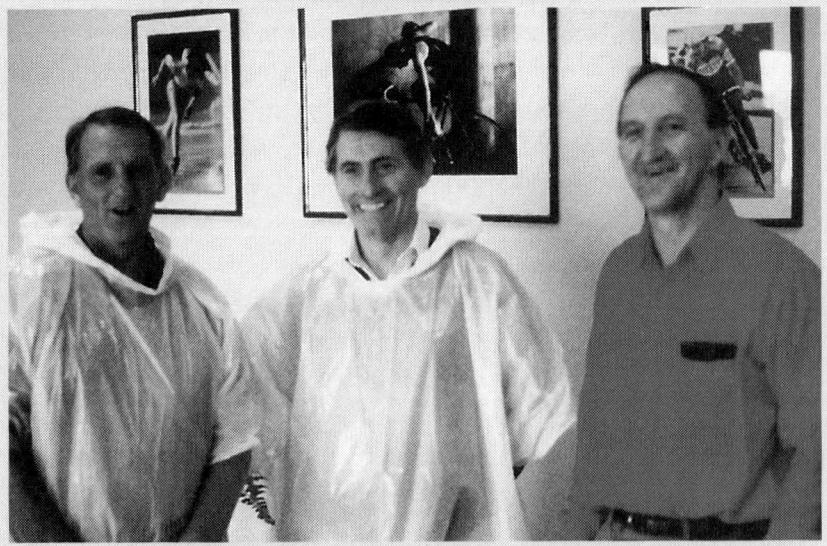

With Brian Sando (centre) and Ken Fitch (right) at a Drugs in Sport meeting. (BRIAN CORRIGAN'S COLLECTION)

'What would I tell athletes about ginseng? ... It is not worth the money.'

39. ALTERNATIVE MEDICINE

ALTERNATIVE MEDICINE WAS once neatly defined as anything used for health care that had not been taught in Medical School. This definition is now long out of date as over the past ten years appropriately trained therapists and medical practitioners have increasingly used it. Many therapies once regarded as 'alternative' now have some legitimate medical role. Sales of alternative medicines in the United States have reached $14 billion a year, and may be used by up to 50 per cent of the American population. In Australia, sales top $3 billion, and are still rising. More and more athletes are also using alternative medicines, looking for a vital competitive edge. They often see their salvation in the use of various so-called 'natural' over-the-counter medications. In America, sale of sports supplements alone now total over $1 billion annually.

Alternative medicine supplements are usually self-prescribed and their users may not consider them as medicines, so that 70 per cent do not bother to mention their use to their GPs. But complications or interactions between a therapeutic medication and a herb can arise. In the United States, 18 per cent of adults use prescription drugs at the same time as their herbal products, and so 15 million Americans are at risk of potential drug–herb interactions.

The alternative medicine industry has major political clout in America and was able to successfully lobby the US Congress to pass an Act that exempts their products from regulation, thus the general population has unlimited access to the 'alternative' drugs, despite a lack of data concerning safety and efficacy, and their vague alleged benefits.

The IOC has repeatedly warned athletes about the problems of taking supplements. 'Natural' is not the same as 'safe'. Contamination with various products, including other medicinal compounds or plants, is well recognised. Products advertised in health magazines may contain unidentified ingredients. Much more research about their use is needed before these treatments could be recommended as standard treatment.

HERBS AND MEDICINAL plants are the most commonly used forms of alternative medicine. Besides promising to promote health, prevent and treat disease, they are also sold to athletes to improve performance. In Australia, ginseng is the most commonly consumed.

In 1989, when the Australian soccer team was in South Korea for a few weeks, some players asked me if they could be treated with ginseng. I told them I did not know enough about it, but would try to do some research on it while we were there. If it turned out to be as good as claimed, they could go on it. The Korean ginseng information centre was most helpful in providing some documents in English, but not the scientific information I was seeking. It did, however, stimulate my interest in ginseng and alternative medicine, an interest I have maintained ever since.

Ginseng has been used in the Far East for some 5000 years as a tonic to revitalise the functioning of the whole organism. It has been touted as a cure for nearly everything from a headache to impotence. One claimed benefit was as an aphrodisiac, although American natives used it as a contraceptive. Ginseng is a herb with a human-like shape, one type of which grows wild in China, but it is also found in Korea, North America and Siberia (although Siberian ginseng is a misnomer as it is a different substance, *Eleutherococcus*).

Although any part of the plant may be used, commercial preparations are usually derived from the root. The ginseng plant, after having grown for up to seven years, is harvested and the root dried and divided into two grades, white or red. White ginseng root is unprocessed and sometimes bleached before being dried. The red ginseng is prepared from the white by various processes such as steaming and is much more popular. It is also expensive since it comprises only about 1 per cent of the total production.

Ginseng dietary supplements are typically made from a powder or extract of the ginseng root. It can be taken as a tablet, capsule, liquid, jelly, boiled and then drunk, tea or tea bags, cream, chewing gum or shampoo. It can even be smoked. In the mid-1990s up to six million Americans were reported to be using these ginseng products. Several major theories have been proposed explaining how it works, including a suggestion that it improves memory and another that it stimulates the immune system or the production of cortisone. Chinese medicine regards it as a harmonising agent to restore Qi, the life force, by increasing the body's resistance to stress or illness and so restoring or rejuvenating the body. There are no recognised medical uses for ginseng, but the World Health Organization supports its use as 'a prophylactic and restorative agent'.

COMPLICATIONS FROM USING ginseng are few, but some problems can be attributed to quality control. Commercial preparations are known to contain a large number of different, not well-defined, substances, varying considerably from plant to plant. The ginseng content also varies widely. Recently, 44 commercial ginseng preparations from 11 countries were examined. No ginseng at all was found in six samples, seven had only a small amount of ginseng, while some samples also contained a stimulant and high levels of pesticides, up to 20 times the safe limit.

Ginseng is sold to athletes for its presumed properties of increasing stamina, performance, and relieving stress. Some ginseng preparations taken by athletes may contain contaminants, which may have been deliberately added, or mixed with other herbs that may contain a stimulant.

In Seoul in 1988, English sprinter Linford Christie took a ginseng product and as his urinary levels of a contained stimulant were not particularly high, he was allowed to keep his silver medal, but after a subsequent test he was banned from running in the relay. Antoinette Bevilacqua came fourth in the high jump at the 1996 Atlanta Olympics, but was disqualified after testing positive for a stimulant present in ginseng. In 1993, a Swedish athlete tested positive after taking a ginseng preparation, which on analysis contained no ginseng but large quantities of a stimulant.

So what would I tell athletes about ginseng? I'd point out how the evidence concerning ginseng's effectiveness is not sufficient to merit its use in trying to improve their physical performance, and much more research is needed before it could be so considered. In other words, it is not worth the money.

'There is a story ... a Florida mother, Mrs Maxwell Rogers, who weighed just 56 kilograms, lifted the back of a 1650-kilogram car that had collapsed on her son when a jack slipped.'

40. SPORTS' EVEREST

SHOW ME A champion sportsman or woman and I'll show you someone striving to do better, a lot better. That burning desire to improve is a major component of the sporting ethos. They will always try to run faster, to swim quicker, to extend the limits of performance. The breaking of records is guaranteed to make headlines in newspapers or to grab TV coverage. And rightly so.

One of the most frequent questions I am asked as a sports medicine doctor is what are the limits of performance, and how far can those limits be extended? The question becomes more frequent in the lead-up to an Olympic Games. This was certainly the case as we waited for the Sydney Olympics. To some extent, the easy answer might be that there is no answer. Nobody could accurately predict just what those limits might turn out to be, just as they cannot foretell the future (although some newspaper astrologists and television clairvoyants may beg to disagree).

There is no logical reason why records could not just keep improving. Nonetheless, no one could run 100 metres in five seconds or run a marathon under an hour. The human body is simply not built to be able to accomplish such unbelievable feats. Of course, we are speaking of a drug-free performance. Swallowing a tablet or 20 may make an athlete run faster or be able to lift greater weights, but the real improvement for the human race can only come about from the individual's natural ability to produce greater performances and then watch as the world tries to better it. World sprinting records did not improve because of Ben Johnson's steroid-fuelled performance in Seoul.

One problem is that predictions over the past 100 years have all become so incredibly wrong in so short a time. The most famous attempt was probably that made by Brutus Hamilton, the well-respected and devoted athletics coach from the University of California who had won a silver medal in the 1920 Olympic decathlon and coached several other Olympic gold medal winners. His first predictions concerning the ultimate limits were made in 1934. They rapidly became outdated, with none lasting more than 30 years. His predictions in 1934 included:

- 100 metres in 10.1 seconds (by 2004 there had been 238 performances under 10 seconds).
- 1500 metres in 3 minutes 44 seconds. Herb Elliott ran 3 minutes 35.6 seconds in 1960.
- High jump of 6 feet 11 inches (2.11 metres). This was equalled by Lester Steers at Los Angeles in 1941 and by the early 1990s taken to 2.45 metres (8 feet) by Cuban Javier Sotomayer.

This only proves there is no future in predicting the future.

Just after World War II, one absolute limit was considered to be running a mile in under 4 minutes. The experts pontificated that the body would not be able to withstand the physiological damage. Some runners came agonisingly close to this magic mark, but the brain rather than the body prevented them from making it. When Roger Bannister ran the mile on 6 May 1954 in 3 minutes 59 seconds, collapsing after the finish, not only was he and the world astounded, it was considered that this time would never be bettered. Yet only 46 days later Australian John Landy became the second to crack the barrier, in 3 minutes 57.9 seconds at Turku, Finland. Two years later, seven runners in the one race went under 3 minutes 51 seconds. In 1999, Moroccan Hicham El Guerrouj, the man who went on to win silver in the 1500 metres at the 2000 Sydney Olympics and the world championship a year later (and again in 2003) ran 3 minutes 43.13 seconds for the mile.

The limits of performance depend on how the body is made and works, but the psychological limits, self-imposed by the human mind —

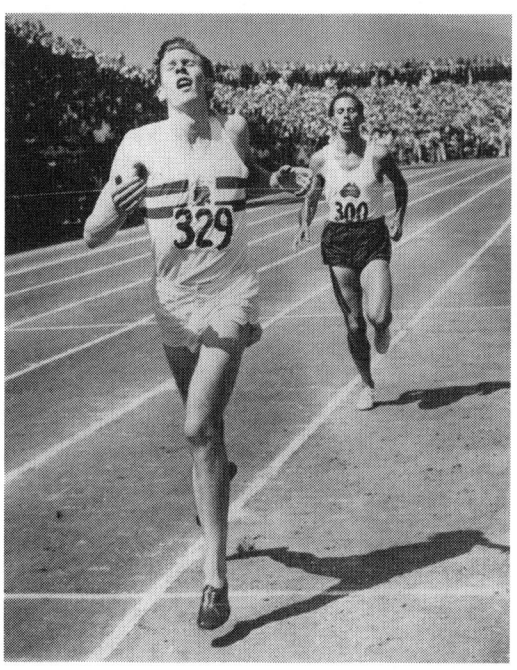

It seemed impossible when Roger Bannister broke the 4-minute mile in May 1954, but the psychological barrier had come down. Just over six weeks later, John Landy did it, too. Here, Bannister leads Landy at the the British Empire Games in Vancouver, BC, in August 1954, the first time two runners finished under 4 minutes. (AAP IMAGE/AP)

may be of even greater importance. It may be these limits are naturally imposed to prevent the body from pushing too far and damaging itself. The occasion, the competition, the crowd, all may contribute to the adrenaline flowing to produce an increased effort. Many stories have been told, and some verified, of incredible feats of strength performed when someone is faced with death. Just one example, there is a story of an incident in 1960 when a Florida mother Mrs Maxwell Rogers, who weighed just 56 kilograms, lifted the back of a 1650 kilogram car that had collapsed on her son when a jack slipped. She suffered multiple fractures in her spine in the effort, but her son was saved.

World records have declined at a steady rate over the past century as each generation improved on the previous one. It has been estimated that there has been an average improvement of 2 per cent in most sports every four years. Accordingly, the graph indicating improvement in human performance has steadily risen. The upward curve demonstrating improvement may be flattening out and in the future may even flatten out appreciably more, but it will still continue upwards, even though changes would be extremely small. Times measured now in thousands of a second may even eventually have to be measured in millionths of a second.

In 1968, the Australian long jump record was a fraction under 8 metres; the Olympics record 8.12 metres (set by Ralph Boston at the 1960 Rome Games); and the world record at 8.35 metres (shared by Boston and Russian Igor Ter-Ovanesyan). American Bob Beamon jumped 8.90 metres in the rarefied air of Mexico City at the 1968 Olympics. At that time, it was thought to be the ultimate. Surely nobody could ever beat that. Yet broken it was, almost equalled in 1987 and surpassed four years later by American Michael Powell (8.95 metres).

In swimming, men and women sprint times have improved at a faster rate than their counterparts on the track. In July 1922, Johnny Weissmuller, (aka Tarzan), became the first person in the world to swim under 1 minute for the 100m freestyle with a time of 58.6 seconds. When the Russian Vladimir Salnikov swam a world record of 14 minutes 58.27 seconds to win gold in the 1500 metres at the 1980 Moscow Olympics, he swam under 1 minute for each of the 15 of his 100-metre splits. Dutch swimmer, Pieter van den Hoogenband swam 47.8 seconds for the 100 metres in Sydney in 2000. I could go on, for there are a host of examples.

When is enough enough?

Enough is never going to be enough. As soon as a record is broken, someone, somewhere will use it as the benchmark to beat sometime in the future.

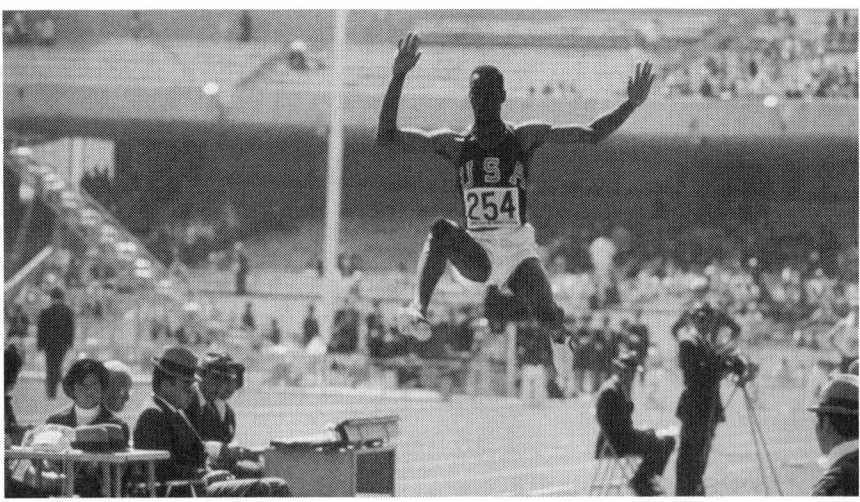

American long jumper Bob Beamon seemed to have performed a miracle at the 1968 Mexico Olympics by jumping 8.9 metres. His record held until 1991 when another American, Michael Powell, jumped 8.95 metres.

(AAP IMAGE/SPORT THE LIBRARY/PRESSE SPORTS)

'John Landy, the first Australian runner to break the four-minute mile barrier, says that on the morning before the race he had a couple of meat pies and an ice-cream sundae.'

41. SEVEN PILLARS OF IMPROVEMENT

SEVEN FACTORS THAT have increased the limits of human performance are worth examining, although it will not be possible to consider them in any depth, for that would require a book of its own. Here are the basics in a nutshell.

1. TECHNOLOGY

Some recent improvements include:

- Better running tracks. Not so long ago athletes ran on cinder tracks, they have since been superseded by the bouncier synthetic tartan surfaces.
- Starting blocks, greatly improved.
- Running shoes are better designed, better made and are lighter.
- Pole vaults have been changed to a fibreglass.
- Bicycles and helmets are now aerodynamically designed to overcome air friction, the cyclist's major problem.
- Archery has changed greatly since the introduction of carbon fibres.

- Better protective gear, high jumpers and pole vaulters now have foam landings; cricketers have worn protective head gear since 1978.
- In swimming, better materials and costume design have helped to minimise friction. Swimming pools are better designed. Rules involving turns have changed, and bigger lane ropes reduce wash.
- Competition has become more intense over recent decades for many reasons, including the Cold War, and the increased amount of money available in sport. The laboratories of the Australian Institute of Sport (AIS), opened in 1981, can now readily measure and study performance factors. Other national sports institutes have been set up, and are producing better coaching and skill enhancement, better medical care and improved and more intensive training methods. The staff at these institutes are also able to disseminate more information, particularly about tactics

2. TECHNIQUES

The development of new techniques owes much to increased and improved training and coaching. All aspects of technique can now be analysed using computer models and biomechanical analysis of most sporting actions and, if need be, improved. Compare this to Australian sprinters in 1956 who trained part-time in summer, with no weight training, and none of the facilities now available.

3. PHYSIOLOGICAL LIMITS

These are most easily demonstrated with an example of contrasting the differences between long distance runners and sprinters.

Long distance runners need to be tall, with relatively long, thin legs but big chests as their body depends on how much oxygen their heart and lungs can supply to the muscles. Their muscle fibres are called white fibres, or 'slow twitch', and are less powerful than red (fast twitch) fibres, but are able to last longer. Fuel for long-distance exercise, be it oxygen or the glucose-storing glycogen, must be supplied as the athlete is running along. When the supply of glycogen is exhausted, the body needs to switch to its alternative energy supply, which is fat. That process is what runners call 'hitting the wall'.

Sprinters, on the other hand, are born not made. They need to be shorter and squatter with a different muscular make-up, comprising of red, 'fast twitch' muscle fibres which are able to contract powerfully and rapidly, but tire more easily. Sprinters can get by without an immediate supply of oxygen, called anaerobic metabolism, but will have to breath more heavily after the race to make up the oxygen difference.

4. PSYCHOLOGICAL FACTORS

The mind plays an essential role in sport. The role of the psychologist in sport was once denigrated — tell a team you intended to introduce a psychologist and they would doubt your own sanity. Times have changed for the better and the psychologist is now considered an essential member of the medical staff in almost all sports. Elite athletes today are placed under great stress and psychologists can do a lot to alleviate it.

Champions have a winner's mindset and the will to win, which the psychologist can tap into to help and develop a positive approach. On the other hand, negative feelings that can prevent athletes from properly utilising their skills can be circumvented. It is worth noting that Wayne Bennett, the renowned coach of the Brisbane Broncos Rugby League team, introduced yoga classes into pre-season training for 2004 as part of his scheme for the players to set aside thoughts of the finish to the 2003 season — the longest losing sequence in the club's history.

These days new techniques, such as brain scans and biofeedback, have also been developed to investigate athletes and their mental conditioning to allow physical improvement.

There was one, somewhat offbeat, method used by the South Korean judo team in Seoul, where they won two gold medals. They would sit meditating for some time. All right, I hear you say, there's nothing unusual about that. Except it was after midnight in a cemetery, and when they returned back they would study tapes of their opponents.

5. NUTRITION

One of the major advances in sports medicine over the past few years has been in the science of sports nutrition. Improved nutrition over recent years has made a substantial contribution to increasing athletes' size and weight, improving athletic performance and helping set new sporting records.

Sports nutritionists and sport nutrition departments that put out valuable information, are now commonplace. It is not so long ago that the pre-competition meal, in all sports, comprised of steak and eggs. John Landy, the first Australian runner to break the four minute mile barrier, says that on the morning before the race he had a couple of meat pies and an ice-cream sundae.

It is no secret that athletes would do anything within legal bounds to get a competitive edge and reduce fatigue. As a result, many use a variety of supplements, although most lack any scientific evidence as to their efficacy, and are commonly hyped with claims that are never substantiated. The most commonly used nutritional supplements, for which some evidence exists concerning their value, include carbohydrate loading, some energy bars, and creatine. (Creatine is an amino acid that plays an essential role in controlling how a muscle works. Its greatest value is in certain types of sporting performances — high intensity, short duration exercise such as sprinting or weightlifting.) With carbohydrates, the timing of its supply to the body may be even more important than other factors.

Enhanced use of fluid replacements has also been a great improvement. Marathon runners used to believe that they should take in no fluids at all during their race, even in hot weather and even when it had been demonstrated that replacing fluid made them more efficient. How wrong they were!

6. POPULATION

The genetic pool for athletic talent expands at a great rate as the world's population increases. More talent may be, or rather has been, discovered, especially in the so-called developing countries. In the West, increased leisure time is among the many social changes, allowing more time to train, practice and perform.

7. GENETICS

There can be no doubt about the importance of genetics, even without putting cricket's Waugh twins or tennis' Williams sisters into the equation, and all the methods mentioned above can be looked on as helping to reach one's genetic potential. The future lies with genetics.

'It is easy to imagine how people in 100 years from now will look back and think of gene technology as we do of alchemy in the Middle Ages.'

42. THE GENIE IN THE BOTTLE

THE KEY TO the future of many of the issues, such as the limits of human performance and the problems of drugs in sport, is linked to genetics. Genetics is the study of heredity, how the various characteristics in all living organisms are inherited. The role of nature versus nurture has long been debated in sports medicine and scientific circles. To what degree heredity plays in determining such factors as body build, lung capacity, heart volume and hand–eye coordination was at best a guess. Published scientific information had produced widely varied data, while deductive methods, including anecdotal evidence and twin studies, were relatively crude.

Recent advances in knowledge about genes and gene therapy have occurred at an unbelievable rate, and are revolutionising the future of medicine. (It might be noted in passing that cloning, another big issue for the future, is a different proposition from gene therapy.)

The huge scientific program known as the Human Genome Project (the word genome is a combination of gene plus chromosome) was completed in the year 2000, five years ahead of schedule. The next big step is to develop a better understanding of, first, how the necessary instructions of genes work and, second, gene therapy.

GENE THERAPY IS certainly the pathway to the future. Its importance in the field of medicine is that a normal gene may be substituted for an abnormal, faulty gene, so that some 4000 different diseases could potentially be cured. The technique for this undertaking is relatively simple. Once the gene has been identified, it is easily injected into the body using some carrier, usually an altered virus whose genes have been replaced with the desired gene.

Sadly, gene therapy is also very much the sports drug of the future, although the problem in sport is really not so much gene therapy as gene doping. It is the greatest problem facing sports medicine today, rendering drug testing as we know it obsolete. It will take many millions, maybe billions, of dollars to provide the technology to combat it. Even then testers will be playing catch-up with drug abusers. It is easy to imagine how people in 100 years from now will look back and think of gene technology now as we do of alchemy in the Middle Ages.

Bigism is a well-recognised condition in America when parents desperately want their children to become tall. To become a basketball player, or president of some large institution, or even President of the United States, being tall has become a necessity.

In the future, it might be possible to order height, just as fruit and vegetables can be ordered on the Internet, by requesting: 'Yes, we'll have enough height for our son (or daughter, as the case may be) to become tall enough to be a basketball player, please.'

Human growth hormone was developed and produced using genetic mechanisms to treat dwarfed children, allowing them to grow to a more normal height. But normal athletes now use it illegally to increases their height and boost strength.

Are you too fat? The genes to control body fat are now known and will soon become available for use.

The type of muscle fibre in muscles is under genetic control. Genes have a large influence on the percentage of fast and slow twitch fibres, muscle size, composition and strength. Gene therapy could determine or alter the type of muscle fibres, increasing muscle bulk, with a large increase in muscular development and strength. Genetically modified fast twitch fibres in individual leg muscles could be targeted for use by sprinters. Alternatively, distance runners could inject a different series of genes to increase the amount of oxygen carried in their blood, and so may improve their times by a large amount. Muscles of all animals process oxygen in a specialised unit within the muscle cells, known as mitochondria. In humans, they make up about 3 per cent of the cell volume. Many animals that run faster than man have much bigger mitochondria. With genetic engineering, humans will also be able to increase the size of their mitochondria.

Blood boosting is another good example. A difficult and cumbersome method to use, athletes found they could obtain the same effect by using EPO, injected three times a week. Better still, the gene responsible for EPO production, already identified by the Human Genome Project, can be injected and the body could become a factory churning out extra EPO. In addition, it will be undetectable by any means now known, as the EPO from the introduced gene will be identical to natural EPO. Other, indirect methods could possibly allow its detection, but not the EPO gene itself.

Treatment of injuries will also be revolutionised. New ligaments and tendons could be grown and then made available for immediate treatment by replacing a ruptured one. But there is no truth in the rumour that ligaments or tendons ruptured in a match could be replaced at half-time and the player will be sent back on the field for the second half.

Gene therapy is going to play a major role in the future, probably even more than many people realise. There will be dangers with its use.

HOW LONG BEFORE gene therapy becomes a major problem in sport? Within a few years at best for there are some athletes out there now experimenting with gene therapy. What should happen is that properly conducted scientific studies be carried out to determine how effective this treatment is and find out what the risk factors and side effects are.

The sporting fraternity has already mounted pressure to provide quick results and the history of drugs in sport shows that athletes have a disarming lack of concern for any health problems.

Problems will inevitably arise with gene therapy. For example, the successful experiments carried out have been mainly in the laboratory using mice or monkeys. The research into whether or not this can be translated into humans is still not available. In addition, the medical applications of gene therapy aimed at curing or preventing disease are still only in their preliminary stages. A great deal more needs to be learnt and understood about how genes work in the body and what will happen after they have been introduced. An injected gene to treat a disease may not necessarily be what is required for an athlete trying to improve some part of his or her body.

Many arguments have surrounded the development of genetically modified food — 'Frankenfood', as it has been called — and concerns will increase dramatically when humans, not plants, are being modified.

Once in the body, it may not then be possible for the body to eliminate a modified gene, unless some sort of bodily switch can be developed. Also, the carrier used to insert the gene into the body is usually an altered virus. Nobody yet knows for certain how the body and the body's immune system will react to such a virus.

The first death resulting from genetic modification was that of Jesse Gelsinger, an 18-year-old man involved in a project at the University of Pennsylvania. He suffered from a rare metabolic disorder controlled by diet and by taking 32 pills a day. Jesse wanted to help in research into the disorder, but 20 hours after the disorder-specific gene was introduced via a weakened cold virus, there was an incredible chain reaction that claimed his life — jaundice, blood-clotting problems, kidney failure, lung failure and brain death.

If the EPO gene is producing excessive amounts of blood cells, the complications will include heart attacks, stroke and death. The gene for growth hormone could continue putting out excess amounts of the hormone, resulting in a disease known as acromegaly, which can be crippling or ultimately fatal.

Many people from different medical and sport medical backgrounds, and also those with a background in law and ethics, will be needed to sort out these questions, not the least being 'Who will fund it?' Already experts are calling it the death of sport as we know it and gene doping is now prohibited in the Olympics.

The problem has become not so much the genie in the bottle. It's whether we are too late and the gene genie has already escaped.

'The awful thing is ... that no one knows who is going to die. The problems are unknown. The possible side effects of so many drugs that athletes *are* taking terrify me.'

43. THG — THE LATEST MENACE

JUST WHEN SOME scientists thought that maybe, just maybe, they had got the scourge of anabolic steroids under control, along came THG (tetrahydrogestrinone). The whole furore exploded in 2003. In June, the United States Anti-Drugs Agency (USADA) received an anonymous tip from a track coach that several top athletes were using an undetectable anabolic steroid. To prove his point, he mailed a syringe containing THG.

All hell broke loose. How long had this been going on? Had Olympic gold medal winners been in on the cheating? Who was behind it? Once the media got hold of the story it was labelled as the biggest drug story since Ben Johnson at Seoul.

THG is a designer steroid almost certainly used by elite sportsmen able to pay the excessive prices being charged on the black market. THG was created from two other known steroids — trenbolone and gestrinone. Trenbolone was known as a reasonably popular steroid. Gestrinone (otherwise known as Dimetriose) was used for treating endometriosis, a common, painful abdominal problem suffered by young women. The chemical modifications made THG undetectable in the usual tests for steroids. Cheating sports stars were able to take the steroid in liquid form by placing it under the tongue, allowing it to be quickly absorbed. This made it a lot more toxic on the liver than injectable anabolic steroids.

The whistleblowing coach claimed the source of THG was a well-known Californian company that was selling it as a nutritional supplement for athletes. American authorities raided the company, court proceedings were instituted and the United States Food and Drug Administration (FDA) quickly banned its use.

Meanwhile, a team under Dr Don Catlin, head of the IOC registered drug testing laboratory at the University of Southern California, received the sample in the syringe. A massive technical effort involving many scientists working day and night for several months first had to identify the THG and then to develop a successful test for it.

It wasn't long before the drug cheats were uncovered.

By mid-November 2003, four American athletes tested positive taken in samples at the US National Championships four months before. European 100 metres champion Dwain Chambers of Britain also tested positive. And four players from the Oakland Raiders in the NFL were caught in the net, but they were not suspended. Incredibly, the NFL Commissioner Paul Tagliabue explained, 'You don't go around changing the traffic sign after I pass. It was a yield sign when I passed, not a stop sign.' Of course, Tagliabue has highlighted the very touchy ethical problem of whether or not retrospective drug tests should be allowed.

Neverthless, swimming's international governing body FINA (Federation Internationale de Natation) decided to re-test all samples collected from swimmers at their 2003 World Championships. Thankfully none of the tests proved positive. Meanwhile the IOC announced it planned to re-test hundreds of samples from the 2002 Salt Lake City Winter Olympics. The IOC president Jacques Rogge went on record as suggesting the anonymous whistleblowing coach should be awarded the Nobel Peace Prize.

'We wouldn't have a test otherwise,' Rogge said.

The last has not been heard of this latest drug problem and its wider implications for the future. The discovery that sportsmen were using THG only happened because someone gave the authorities the drug. Not only does no one know if it works, but no one knows who is going to die. The problems are unknown. The possible side effects of so many drugs that athletes *are* taking terrify me.

By sports' very nature, we're always playing catch-up, and we always will be. We don't know how many other drugs are out there. No one knows.